AF614796

Ventricular Geometry in Post-Myocardial Infarction Aneurysms

V Rao Parachuri • Srilakshmi M. Adhyapak

Ventricular Geometry in Post-Myocardial Infarction Aneurysms

Implications for Surgical Ventricular Restoration

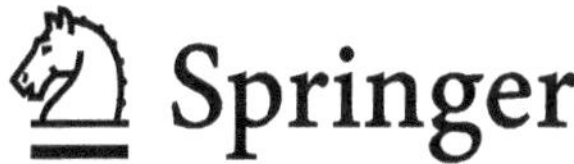

Authors
V Rao Parachuri
Department of Cardiothoracic Surgery
Narayana Hrudayalaya
Bangalore
India

Srilakshmi M. Adhyapak
Department of Cardiology
St. John's Medical College Hospital
Bangalore
India

ISBN 978-1-4471-2860-1 ISBN 978-1-4471-2861-8 (eBook)
DOI 10.1007/978-1-4471-2861-8
Springer Dordrecht Heidelberg New York London

Library of Congress Control Number: 2012939724

Printed on acid-free paper

Springer is part of Springer Science+Business Media (www.springer.com)

This book is dedicated to all the scientists, researchers, students, anatomists, physiologists, cardiologists, and cardiac surgeons who have dedicated their lives to the evolution of innovations to tackle and reverse the relentless downhill course of the syndrome of heart failure.

Foreword

This book by a cardiac surgeon and a cardiologist offers a detailed analysis of ventricular function at the cellular, hemodynamic, and clinical levels with a review of surgical procedures that have historically been aimed at surgical restoration of the distorted left ventricle to its more normal volume and ellipsoid configuration following myocardial infarction or dilated cardiomyopathy. Some of these patients may be candidates for heart transplantation, but many are not, and can benefit by a conventional surgical approach. It is a fascinating story. The early work of Dor, Jatene, Cooley, and others is carefully evaluated, and Parachuri's own modification of surgical ventricular restoration is documented (with a complementary video) with late follow-up and objective assessment. Dr. Parachuri has performed over 800 ventricular endopatch procedures clinically, and this experience provides a significant clinical foundation for the authors' recommendations of advanced surgical correction (therapeutic remodeling) of scarred and aneurysmal left ventricles. It is a clinical experience which is unlikely to be duplicated currently in North America, given the frequency of interventional reflow procedures and thrombolysis that appear to have significantly reduced the incidence of mechanical complications of myocardial infarction. Nevertheless, the experience and recommendations made in this book are applicable to all current populations who experience heart failure. This book also includes assessment of concomitant coronary bypass grafting, mitral valve procedures, and treatment of ventricular arrhythmias.

I had the good fortune of working with Dr. Parachuri at St. Vincent Hospital in Worcester, MA, in the 1990s. Even then his skills as a cardiac surgeon predicted a bright future, manifested in this carefully documented book on the assessment and surgical treatment of heart failure. This book will serve well the interests of cardiothoracic surgical residents, cardiologists in training, as well as practicing clinicians in cardiac disease and serious students of cardiac function and failure.

Willard M. Daggett, M.D.

Preface

The goal of this book is to provide cardiac surgeons and cardiologists a definitive perspective of optimal surgical ventricular restoration in patients with advanced heart failure due to large ventricular aneurysms following transmural myocardial infarctions. The recently concluded STICH multicenter randomized trial has vitiated the role of surgical reshaping of the dilated, distorted ventricle in patients ineligible for cardiac transplantation. This mechanical complication of transmural myocardial infarctions leading to intractable and refractory heart failure is a persisting entity in both the developed and developing countries of the world. The continuing occurrence of this devastating complication is due to a conundrum of logistic constraints restraining timely revascularization and certain ethnic predisposing factors peculiar to certain specific populations. This opens the avenue for rethinking about the surgical techniques involved in the palliation of this condition. Therefore, surgical ventricular restoration of these adversely remodeled ventricles has a continuing role in the management of this difficult subset of patients. The process of cardiac remodeling has been studied extensively, and recent surgical techniques for ventricular restoration have proven late adverse remodeling.

The objective of this book therefore is to discuss the surgical technical evolutions toward a near-ellipsoid ventricular shape which results in near-physiological hemodynamics evident at long term. With our limited objective, this book does not claim to be a compendium or handbook of current information on the selected topics nor is it a review of literature. It is largely the works of the editors and their associates with a balanced point of view. We wish to express our thanks to all the authors and publishers who permitted us to quote their publications, figures, and data in this book. We wish to specially thank Dr. M.R. Girinath at Apollo Hospitals, Chennai, and Dr. Devi Prasad Shetty at Narayana Hrudayalaya Institute of Medical Sciences, Bangalore, for their encouragement.

Finally, we wish to thank the editorial and production staffs of Springer for their professional help and cooperation in producing this book.

Bangalore, India

V Rao Parachuri
Srilakshmi M. Adhyapak

Contents

Anatomy of the Myocardium in the Normal Left Ventricle

1

Introduction

There are several limitations in the understanding of the pathophysiology of heart failure and in defining therapeutic strategies for the same. This is a result of existing lacunae in the understanding of the normal structure and function of the heart in vivo, as well as the molecular and genetic factors influencing crucial steps toward altered geometry and function. Despite the presence of regional inhomogeneity in the normal left ventricle during systole and diastole, a highly effective global function is maintained. This is due to its structural and functional anisotropy.

Normal Left Ventricular Myocardial Geometry

Prolate Ellipsoid Shape of the Left Ventricle

The normal left ventricular shape is a prolate ellipsoid with its long axis directed from apex to base [1]. Hutchins and coworkers [2] studied the shape of the LV in normal individuals by contrast ventriculography. The shape of the LV was defined as prolate ellipsoid, as it conformed to the shape of an ellipse, but was not identical with that of an ellipse. The left ventricular shape should sub serve its optimal function. It should be such that it can eject about 60% of its volume in systole, reduce energy loss at pressure gradients, and its cross-sectional dimensions in systole and diastole should be similar to the sizes of its inlet and outlet ports respectively. As the energy used in the cardiac cycle is the sum of diastolic filling, systolic emptying and a constant for maintenance of the mass of muscle and contained blood, the most efficient ventricular topography should be a compromise between a spherical diastole-determined shape and a conical systole-determined configuration. This range of shapes constitutes at one end of the spectrum the sphere and at the other end an elongated almost conical cigar-shaped structure. Hutchins and coworkers while studying human hearts determined the maximal internal diameter of the left ventricle as 3.1 cm in systole and 5.6 cm in diastole (ratio 1:1.8), compared with an aortic valve diameter of 2 cm and a mitral valve diameter of 3 cm (ratio 1:1.5). The apex to base length of its cavity averages 9.9 cm in systole and 10.7 cm in diastole. In the hearts studied, average left ventricular volume decreased from 153 to 62 mL from diastole to systole, which corresponded to an ejection fraction of 60%. By substituting normal values for maximal LV diameter (d) at the base, and apex to base length (h) into the formula for the volume of a prolate ellipsoid, namely, $V=\pi/6d^2h$, they obtained 50 mL in systole (observed end-systolic volume on ventriculography by Dodge formula was 62 mL) and 176 mL in diastole (observed end-diastolic volume was 153 mL). The mathematical model of an ellipse was therefore considered fairly accurate in defining left ventricular shape.

This shape, however, is subject to several changes during the cardiac cycle. A dimension-

V R. Parachuri, S.M. Adhyapak, *Ventricular Geometry in Post-Myocardial Infarction Aneurysms*,
DOI 10.1007/978-1-4471-2861-8_1,

less shape index was defined by Gibson and Brown. The shape index was 4π(area)/(perimeter)^2 which had a maximum value of 1, or 100% when the cavity was circular in diastole and a minimum of 0 when cavity obliteration occurred in systole. This shape index was therefore the volume enclosed by unit surface area of ventricular wall, allowing quantification of cavity shape changes independent of changes in area and long axis, and its magnitude during ventricular filling and ejection. The systolic reduction in cavity is mediated by a change in shape toward a less circular configuration as well as by reduction in perimeter, both of which occur concomitantly. During diastole, the mechanism of change in cavity area is reverse to that in systole. Throughout the cardiac cycle, the rates of wall movement are similar in all regions of the ventricle. This shape change has a clear functional significance, since in its absence similar reduction in perimeter would lead to a smaller change in area. When extrapolated to ventricular volume, it shows that in the absence of shape change, stroke volume would be reduced by approximately one-third.

Inflow and Outflow of the Left Ventricle

The left ventricular inflow and outflow are at 30° to each other, i.e., "V" shaped. The inlet (mitral valve) and outlet (aortic valve) of the ventricular chamber are in continuity, being separated by a thin membrane—the anterior mitral leaflet. Hence, blood enters and leaves through virtually the same orifice, which makes its flow through the left ventricle bidirectional. The blood flows vertically into the left ventricle through the mitral valve and is propelled out of the left ventricle in the same vertical but opposite direction through the aortic valve, which is continuous with the mitral valve (Fig. 1.1). The left ventricle acts by its unique fiber orientation as a pump to propel blood flow in the reverse direction to its inflow. This bidirectional flow in the left ventricle is required to generate a systolic blood pressure of 120 mmHg in order to propel blood flow to the cranium and through the entire systemic circulation. The ellipsoid shape is crucial for normal ventricular function, which is an adaptation to evolution and assumption of an erect habitus. The amphibian has a spherical ventricle, man has an ellipsoid systemic ventricle, and a giraffe has an extreme ellipsoid (almost cylindrical) ventricle which is required to generate a systolic blood pressure of 300 mmHg with its head erect (Fig. 1.2).

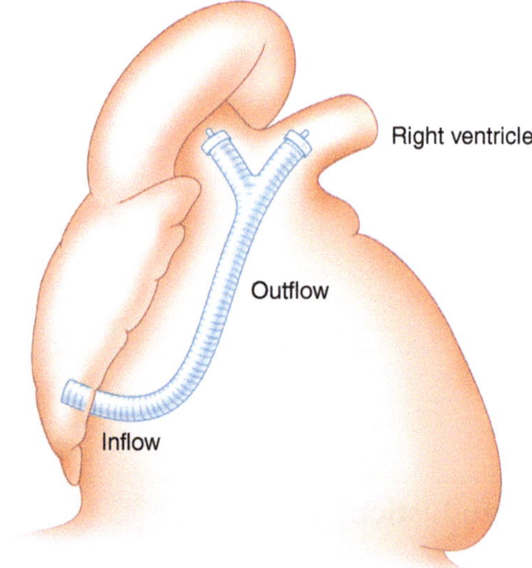

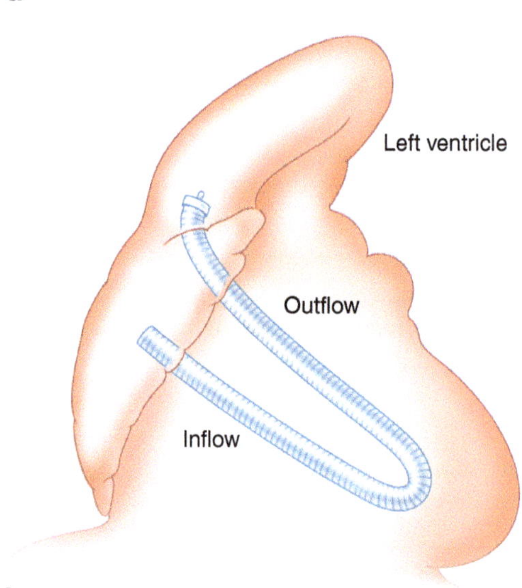

Fig. 1.1 Representation of the in flow and out flow tracts in the right ventricle (**a**) and left ventricle (**b**). *I* Inflow, *O* Outflow

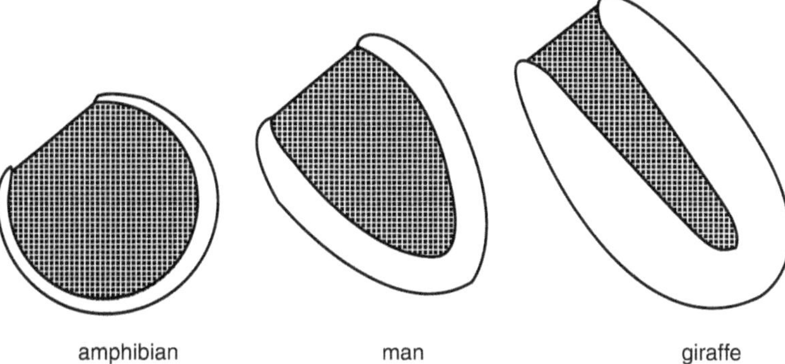

Fig. 1.2 Comparison of the shape (architecture) of the amphibian, human, and giraffe left ventricle. Amphibian LV represents Romanesque (*circular*) architecture of dilated failing heart, contrasted with the Gothic (*elliptical*) healthy human LV and the "extreme Gothic" giraffe LV capable of generating systolic pressures of 300 mmHg routinely (With permission from Coghlan and Hoffman [23]. Copyright Elsevier)

Inflow and Outflow of the Right Ventricle

The right ventricle propels blood into the low pressure pulmonary circulation. Hence, it does not require propulsion at high pressures. A peak systolic pressure of 25 mmHg is necessary for adequate pulmonary blood flow. The inflow and outflow of the right ventricle are at 90° to each other; the tricuspid valve and pulmonary valves in the right ventricle are perpendicular to each other. The blood flows into the right ventricle through the tricuspid valve and flows out through the pulmonary valve, making the blood flow unidirectional (Fig. 1.1). In the right ventricle, the longitudinal fibers are more abundant, and their contraction constitutes a milking effect which propels blood flow through the tricuspid valve and out of the pulmonary valve which are separated by the muscular conus tissue. This flow is linear and is hence termed unidirectional.

Variations in the Normal Left Ventricular Walls and Cavity

The law of Laplace [3, 4] can be used to explain the great variation in thickness of the ventricular wall. In the portions which are very curved (small radius of curvature) as at the apex, the walls though thin can still produce sufficient tension during contraction, to develop enough pressure in the contents. Hence, the apex functions as a fulcrum for cardiac contraction and relaxation. When the wall is relatively less curved as at the base (large radius of curvature), the tension developed must be much greater to produce the same pressure. Hence, the wall should be and is correspondingly thicker. Its free wall is thickest and has the greatest curvatures in both the transverse and apex to base directions. The right ventricular free wall is thinnest but has curvatures only slightly less than that of the left ventricular free wall. The interventricular septum has smaller curvatures and is slightly less thick than the left ventricular free wall. The curve of the septum is such that it usually functions as a component of the left ventricle. The, the posterolateral wall is thicker than the interventricular septum. The transition in thickness is gradual from base to apex.

Left Ventricular Myofiber Anatomy

A knowledge of the orientation of its muscle fibers is vital in understanding its complex function (Fig. 1.3). The descriptions of myocardial architecture have ranged from laminated sheets, layered fibers, and complex nested syncytium to a unique band-like arrangement. The syncytium of

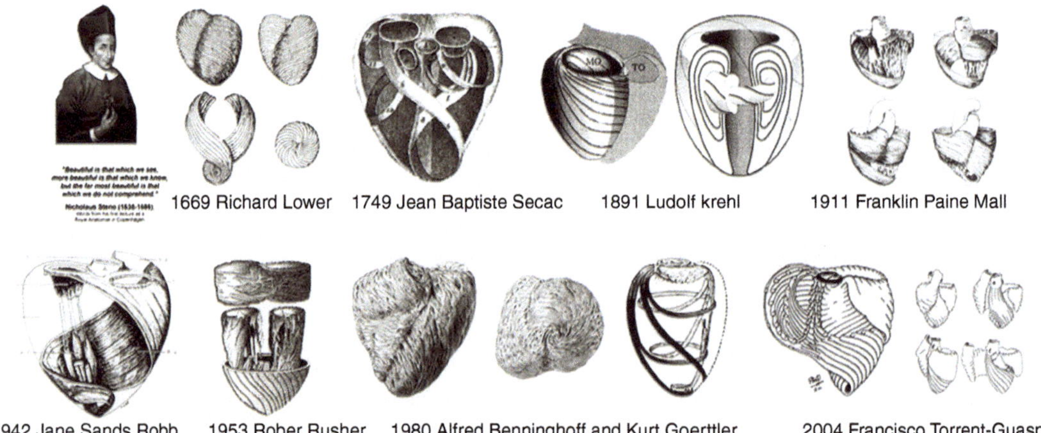

Fig. 1.3 Illustrated historical timetable of the major contributions in understanding the ventricular myocardial architecture (With permission from Coghlan and Hoffman [23]. Copyright Elsevier)

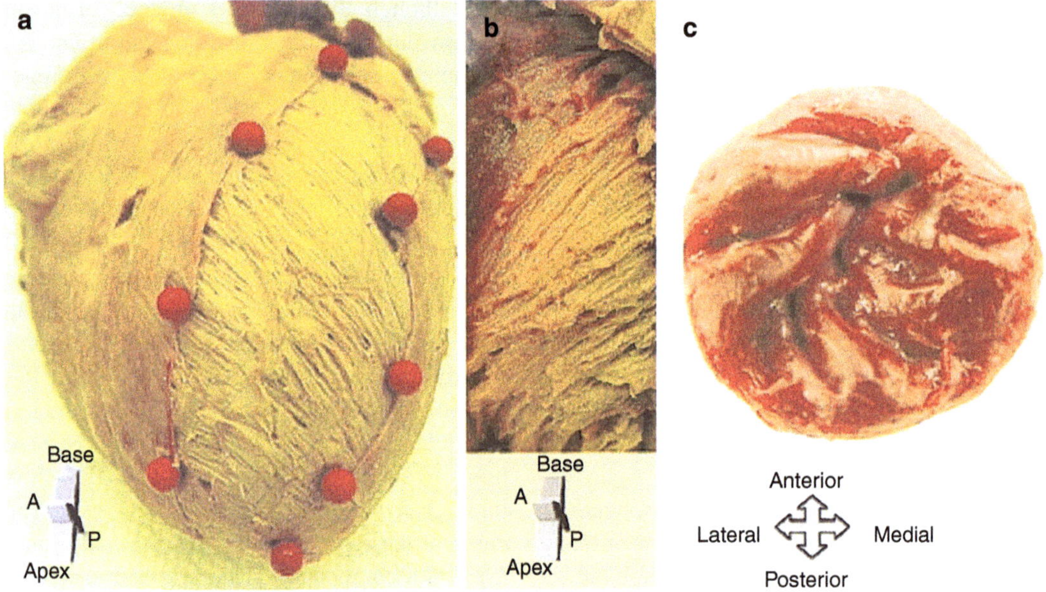

Fig. 1.4 Helical arrangement of muscle fibers in the left ventricle of an explanted adult porcine heart. The arrangement of muscle fibers as seen in the circumferential-longitudinal plane changes from a left-handed helix in the subepicardium (**a**) to a right-handed helix in the subendocardium (**b**). The helical arrangement of the endocardial region is also reflected in the arrangement of trabeculae near the apex (**c**). *A* anterior, *P* posterior (With permission from Sengupta et al. [24])

myocytes is organized into branching laminar sheets, which are approximately four cells thick and roughly stacked from apex to base. A network of extracellular collagen fibers provides tight coupling of myocytes within the sheet and looser coupling between adjacent sheets. Potential spaces between laminae give rise to "cleavage planes" in long- and short-axis sections of the heart (Fig. 1.4). These planes exhibit substantial transmural and regional variations in orientation. These planes constitute the sheet angles in their respective axes. The ventricular myocardium is made up of three layers or laminae which have been established by the elegant studies of Flett and coworkers [5].

Superficial Layer

This is formed by the oblique fibers which course in two separate sheets from the base and are inserted around the apex. They form a twin helix around the ventricle, and during systole and diastole, they cause a wringing effect on the contents of the ventricle, thereby facilitating optimal ventricular filling and emptying. Some of the oblique fibers course on the posterior surfaces of both ventricles, over the anterior surface of the right ventricle, and are inserted at the apex on the anterior surface of the left ventricle. At the apex, the cleavage plane orientation changes from nearly radial at the epicardium to nearly longitudinal at the endocardium. At the base, the cleavage planes are in the opposite direction from that at the apex.

Middle Layer

These are circumferential muscle bundles, cylindrical in shape, and constitute the upper two-thirds of the left ventricular wall. They course downward and forward in the interventricular septum, and turning upward get inserted into the mitral ring. Posteriorly, the circumferential fibers course horizontally from the mitral and tricuspid valve rings. They are mainly located in the mid-wall at the base substantially closer to the epicardium.

Deep Layer

The upper deep layer is thin, and the lower layer is composed of all three muscle fiber types, oblique, circumferential, and longitudinal fibers. The longitudinal fibers course from the mitral ring at the base to the apex.

Torrent-Guasp and coworkers [6, 7] proposed a model where the continuum of myocardial architecture was depicted as a muscle band that was organized spatially into two distinct helicoids, extending from beneath the pulmonary valve across the septum, to beneath the aortic valve (Fig. 1.5). Some authors [8–10] do not agree with this concept of a single helical muscle band. Several studies (autopsy and tagged MRI) [11–13, 20, 21] have proved that the LV comprises of two helical fiber geometries, which are continuous. The base and upper septum have more circumferential fibers, and from mid-wall to apex, the fibers run obliquely.

The oblique fibers have a helical orientation, a right-handed helix in the subendocardium which gradually changes to a left-handed helix in the subepicardium. Mathematical models have proved that the counterdirectional helix is energetically efficient and equalizes redistribution of stress and strain during the cardiac cycle [12, 14]. Incidentally, the counterdirectional arrangement of muscle fibers in the left ventricle mirrors the structural theme that exists for propulsion in other organ systems, such as the alimentary tract, in which the smooth muscles in two opposite directions generate peristaltic waves. Streeter and coworkers [14] introduced the term of helix and transverse angles for quantification of fiber orientation. The helix angle represents the angle between the circumferential axis and the projection of that fiber onto the circumferential-longitudinal plane. The myofiber helix angle changes continuously from the subendocardium to the subepicardium, from a right- to a left-handed helix typically ranging from +60° at the subendocardium to −60° at the subepicardium. The transverse angle represents the angle between the circumferential axis and the projection of myofiber orientation onto the radial-circumferential plane and ranges between −20° and +20° [15, 16, 17]. This change in helix angle is due to the three-dimensional sheet architecture of the myofibers (Fig. 1.6).

Anatomical Understanding of the Extramyocardial Scaffold

The extracellular collagen matrix of the myocardium is an important scaffold in maintaining muscle fiber alignment, ventricular shape and size. It forms a spiral fibrillar structure of endomysial collagen to support a spatial distribution of myocytes and myofibers that ensheaths the adjacent three-dimensional reciprocal spiral arrangement pattern of muscle structure.

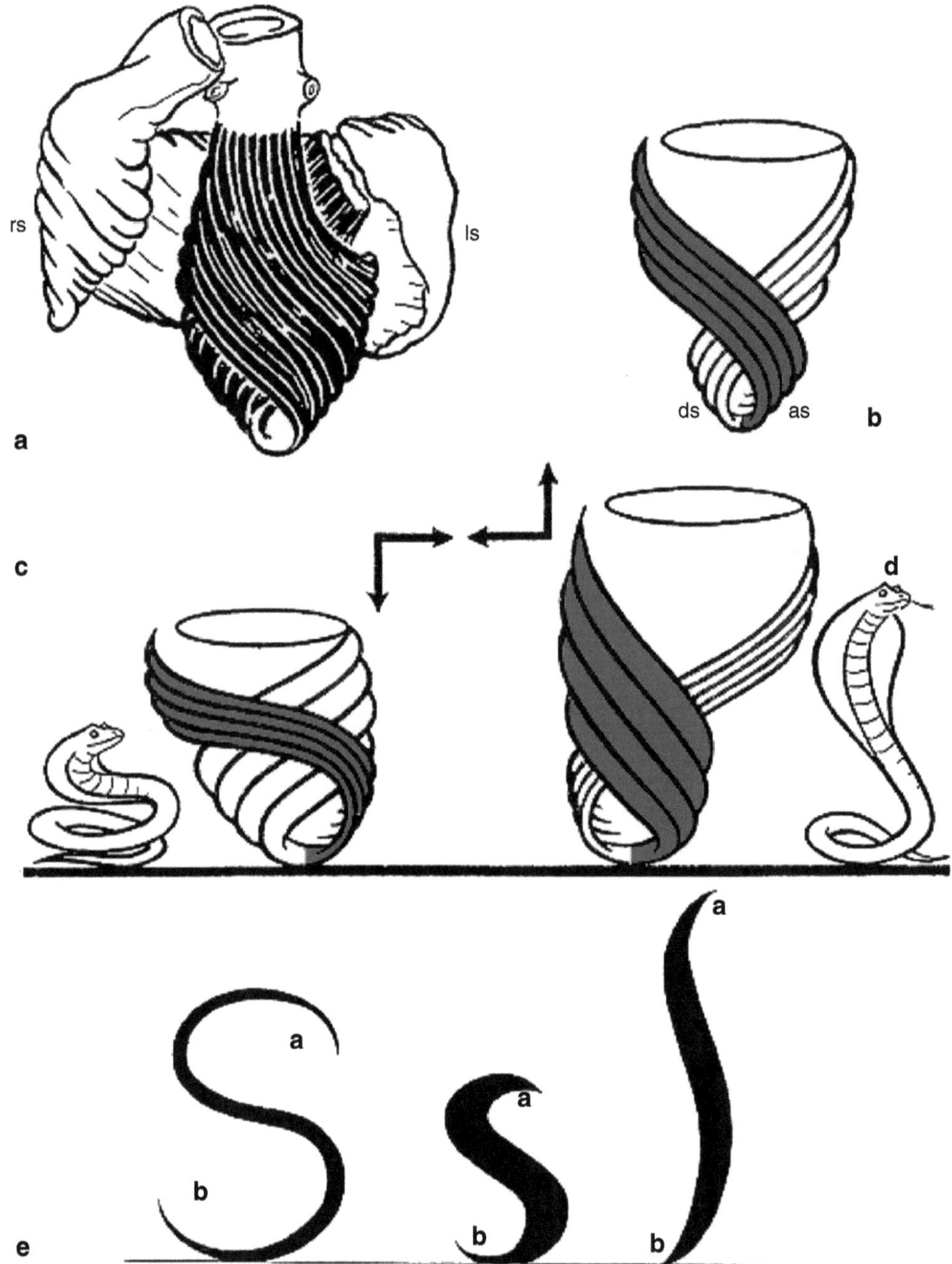

Fig. 1.5 Proposed explanation of the late systolic upward motion of hte base of the ventricles. (**a**) The outer shell formed by the basal loop has been unwound to display the descending and ascending segments of the band, which are seen shaded in (**b–d**) illustrate the way the descending and ascending segments behave during systole. In early systole the base of the heart is pulled toward the apex because of contraction of the descending segment (*thick bundles shaded lightly*); such a movement forces the ascending segment to adopt an "S" configuration in late systole. Contraction of the ascending segment (*thick bundles in light gray*) stiffens such a segment and results in upward movement of the base of the heart. The latter movement could be compared to the way contraction of the dorsal musculature of the snake elongates its body through stiffening of the muscles. Depicted in (**e**) is a scheme of the forced "S" configuration of the ascending segment (*left*), the contraction leads to a shortened "s" (*middle*), and the likely configuration it adopts in late systole (*right*). Contraction of the descending and ascending fibers also results in a rotational motion of the heart, as illustrated in the two intermediate figures, which depict such movement as seen from the apex. (With permission from Francisco Torrent-Guasp et al. [25])

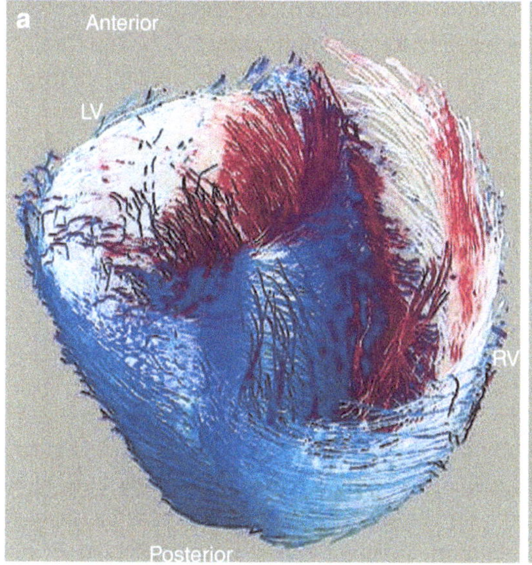

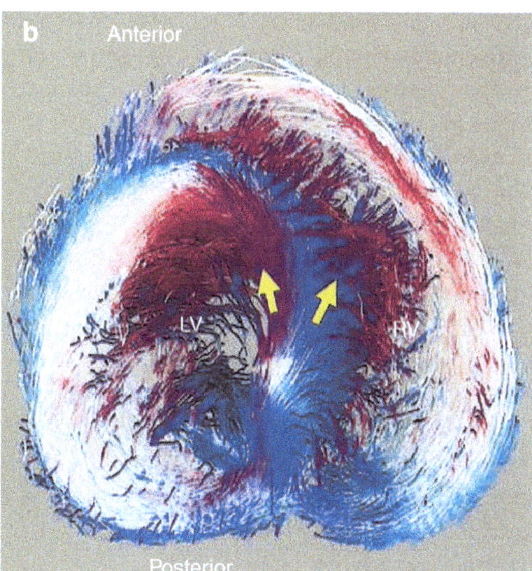

Fig. 1.6 Assessment of cardiac muscle fiber orientation by diffusion tensor magnetic resonance imaging. (*Arrows*) denote the helical fibre orientation at the apex during the cardiac cycle. In these examples (**a** and **b**), scalar and tensor glyph visualization methods have been used to investigate the helical structure of the heart muscle in an explanted fixed canine heart. Right-handed helical orientation (subendocardium) is shown in shades of *purple*, and left-handed helical muscle fiber orientation (subepicardium) is shown in shades of *blue*. The cross-sectional view (**b**) has been viewed from the basal end of the left ventricle (Reproduced from Sengupta et al. with permission). *LV* left ventricle, *RV* right ventricle (With permission from Sengupta et al. [24])

Three-Dimensional Sheet Architecture of Myofibers

The myofibers are arranged in sheet-like structures, which help in cardiac contraction and relaxation [18, 22]. There are three standard cardiac axes which are used to define the three standard cardiac planes: long axis, radial axis, and tangential axis. The three cardiac planes are: radial-longitudinal plane, transverse plane, and the tangential plane. Sheets have a separate local orthogonal coordinate system defined by the fiber orientation axis, the sheet normal axis, and a second axis lying in the sheet plane. In general terms, sheet angles relate the local sheet coordinate system to the standard cardiac coordinate system. The sheet angles have been described by the diffusion tensor MRI.

β' sheet angle ($-90° \leq \beta' \leq \pm 90°$): The angle the sheet makes in the longitudinal-radial plane. It is the angle between the transverse plane and the projection of the secondary eigenvector onto the longitudinal-radial plane. Positive angles rise to the heart base from endocardium to epicardium (or LV endocardium to RV endocardium).

β'' sheet angle ($-90° \leq \beta'' \leq \pm 90°$): The angle the sheet makes in the transverse plane. This is the angle between the longitudinal-radial plane and the projection of the secondary eigenvector onto the transverse plane.

βS-sheet angle ($-90° \leq \beta'' \leq \pm 90°$): The angle between the radial axis and the secondary eigenvector lying in the sheet plane. Positive angles rise to the heart base from endocardium to epicardium.

Embryological Basis of the Myocardial Fiber Orientation

Unlike the mature heart, the embryonic heart grows by hyperplasia. The repetitive interaction of the responses of the ventricular walls to diastolic and systolic pressure, tension and curvature-thickness interrelations produce the cardiac configuration. During cardiogenesis, ventricular diastolic filling induces a spherical configuration analogous to two soap bubbles in contact. The myocytes that generate the most tension are the ones that grow and replicate to the greatest extent, leading to a selection for myocytes that are oriented so as to generate the most systolic tension. The myofibers responsible for reducing cavity size and generate most tension are mid-mural and oriented transversely around the ventricle. These transverse muscle bundles constitute the major portion of wall thickness of the left ventricle. Thus, in the growing ventricle, proliferation of fibers oriented around the more curved circular transverse section is favored by the greater pressure produced by these myocytes in comparison with the less curved apex to base oriented fibers which generate less tension. The final ventricular configuration must therefore represent an interaction of the diastolic passive acquisition of soap-bubble-like curvatures of the three septa, and the systolic induced active growth of myocytes to generate a uniform pressure throughout the variously curved segments of the ventricle.

The helical arrangement of myofibers is evident at a very early stage of cardiac development and can be accelerated or delayed by manipulating the loading conditions. At the embryonic stage, the primitive tubular heart develops from two layers of epithelial cells. The inner layer proliferates and grows toward the ventricular cavity as sheets and chords that develop into trabeculae. Cells in the outer layer proliferate and undergo progressive compaction in response to the functional needs of the growing embryo. The early embryonic heart responds to changes in its mechanical environment. In the presence of pressure overload, there is increased thickening of trabeculae and precocious spiraling of trabecular architecture. The propulsion of blood in the embryonic heart is not due to peristalsis but due to dynamic suction of the tubular heart. Following initial contractions, cardiac looping occurs which promotes a change from the propulsive movements of the tubular heart to the twisting torsional movements seen in adult life. The progressive addition of outer compact spiral layers contributes to the efficiency of ejection and suction in the developing heart.

The double helix is embryologic in origin [7, 19]. The reasons for the differences in orientation of the subendocardial helix and subepicardial helix can be seen in the embryology of the myocardium. The first region of differentiation of myoblasts into striated fibers is in the epicardium. They have an obliquely horizontal orientation. The LV empties laterally into the right ventricle through the interventricular canal in utero. The fibers are parallel to the path of ejection. Weiss and coworkers [19] demonstrated that cell lines are laid parallel to the direction of mechanical tension applied. The inner fibers are laid when the LV has developed considerably; that is, as it becomes larger, the interventricular canal becomes smaller and the aorta becomes the main pathway of ejection. The endocardial helix is therefore in a different direction from the epicardial helix.

Thus, the left ventricular architecture is uniquely different from the right ventricle, as it is equipped with oblique myofibers which serve the mechanism of torsion for effective LV filling and emptying.

References

1. Rankin JS, McHale PA, Arentzen CE, Ling D, Greenfield Jr JC, Andersen RW. The three dimensional dynamic geometry of the left ventricle in the conscious dog. Circ Res. 1976;39:304–13.
2. Hutchins GM, Brawley RK. Shape of the human cardiac ventricles. Am J Cardiol. 1978;41:646–54.
3. Burton AC. The importance of the shape and size of the heart. Am Heart J. 1957;54:801–10.
4. Wong YK, Rautaharju PM. Stress distribution within the left ventricular wall approximated as a thick ellipsoid shell. Am Heart J. 1968;5:649–62.
5. Flett RL. The musculature of the heart, with its application to physiology, and a note on heart rupture. J Anat. 1928;62:439–75.
6. Torrent-Guasp FF, Ballester M, Buckberg GD. Spatial orientation of the ventricular muscle band: physiologic contribution and surgical implications. J Thorac Cardiovasc Surg. 2001;122:389–92.
7. Sedemera D. Form follows function: developmental and physiological view on ventricular myocardial architecture. Eur J Cardiothorac Surg. 2005;28: 526–8.

8. Criscione JC, Rodrigues F, Miller DC. The myocardial band: simplicity can be a weakness. Eur J Cardiothorac Surg. 2005;28:363–4.
9. Andersen RH, Ho SY, Redmann K, Sanchez-Quintana D, Lunkenheimer PP. The anatomical arrangement of the myocardial cells making up the ventricular mass. Eur J Cardiothorac Surg. 2005;28:517–25.
10. Chen J, Liu W, Zhang H. Regional ventricular wall thickening reflects changes in cardiac fiber and sheet structure during contraction: quantification with diffusion tensor MRI. Am J Physiol Heart Circ Physiol. 2005;289:H1898–907.
11. Vendelin M, Bovedeerd PH, Engelbrechet J, Arts T. Optimising ventricular fibers: uniform strain or stress, but not ATP consumption, leads to high efficiency. Am J Physiol Heart Circ Physiol. 2002;283: H1072–81.
12. Nielsen PM, Le Grice IJ, Smaill BH, Hunter PJ. Mathematical model of geometry and fibrous structure of the heart. Am J Physiol. 1991;260:H1365–78.
13. Grider JR. Reciprocal activity of longitudinal and circular muscle during intestinal peristaltic reflex. Am J Physiol Gastrointest Liver Physiol. 2003;284: G768–75.
14. Streeter Jr DD, Spotniz HM, Patel DP, Ross Jr J, Sonnenblick EH. Fiber orientation in the canine left ventricle during diastole and systole. Circ Res. 1969; 24:339–47.
15. Geertz L, Bovendeerd P, Nicolay K, Arts T. Characterisation of the normal cardiac myofiber in goat measured with MR diffusion tensor imaging. Am J Physiol Heart Circ Physiol. 2002;283:H139–45.
16. Greenbaum RA, Ho SY, Gibson DG, Becker AE, Andersen RH. Left ventricular fiber architecture in man. Br Heart J. 1981;45:248–63.
17. Grant RP. Notes on the muscular architecture of the left ventricle. Circulation. 1965;32:301–8.
18. Gilbert HS, Benson AP, Li P, Holden AV. Regional localization of left ventricular sheet structure: integration with current models of cardiac fiber, sheet and band structure. Eur J Cardiothorac Surg. 2007;32: 231–49.
19. Weiss P. Mechanical tension and fiber orientation in cultures of fibroblasts. Arch Entwicklungsmech Organ. 1929;116:438.
20. Takayama Y, Costa KD, Covell JW. Contribution of laminar myofiber architecture to load dependent changes in mechanics of LV myocardium. Am J Physiol Heart Circ Physiol. 2002;282:H1510–20.
21. Costa KD, Takayama Y, McCulloch AD, Covell JW. Laminar fiber architecture and three dimensional systolic mechanics in canine ventricular myocardium. Am J Physiol Heart Circ Physiol. 1999;276:H595–607.
22. Moore CC, McVeigh ER, Elias A. Quantitative tagged magnetic resonance imaging of the normal human ventricle. Top Magn Reson Imaging. 2000;11(6): 359–71.
23. Coghlan C, Hoffman J. Leonardo da Vinci's flights of the mind must continue: cardiac architecture and the fundamental relation of form and function revisited. Eur J Cardiothorac Surg. 2006;29:S4–17.
24. Sengupta PP, Korinek J, Belohlavek M. Left ventricular structure and function basic science for cardiac imaging. J Am Coll Cardiol. 2006;48:1988–2001.
25. Francisco Torrent-Guasp, Manel Ballester, Gerald D. Buckberg, Francesc Carreras, Albert Flotats, Ignasi Carrió, Ana Ferreira, Louis E. Samuels, Jagat Narula. Spatial orientation of the ventricular muscle band: Physiologic contribution and surgical implications. J Thorac Cardiovasc Surg. 2001;122:389–392.

Normal Left Ventricular Dynamics: Contraction and Relaxation Patterns

2

Introduction

The left ventricular function follows its form. The uniqueness of its myofiber arrangement defines its unique function. As implied in the previous chapter, its inflow and outflow are literally continuous, making the filling and ejection of blood bidirectional through literally two orifices which are in anatomical continuity. For this to occur, the left ventricle has to adopt a "wringing" effect of torsion in clockwise and counterclockwise directions. This is an evolutionary adaptation to assumption of the erect posture by man. The function of torsion during systole and diastole is mediated by the oblique myocardial fibers which are unique to the left ventricle. In this chapter, we discuss the patterns of ventricular systole and diastole throughout the cardiac cycle. This understanding is crucial to grasp the perturbations occurring in heart failure, in modulating the therapies for amelioration of the same.

Normal Left Ventricular Deformation During the Cardiac Cycle

Nuclear magnetic resonance tagging with 3D MRI enables noninvasive tracking throughout the LV myocardium during the cardiac cycle [1]. The contributions of myocyte diameter and sliding between bundles of myocytes or myocyte laminae to myocardial wall thickening have been studied. The changes in fiber thickness alone could not account for the changes in myocardial thickness during systole. The "cleavage planes" between groups of myocytes also played a significant role in systole and diastole. The sliding of myofibers as permitted by the "cleavage planes" between them was an important mechanism in cardiac contraction. This was evidenced by the "cleavage planes" having a more vertical alignment in diastole and a more horizontal alignment in systole. The laminar structure of the myocardium is critical for normal ventricular dynamics. In addition to sliding, the sheets participate in myocardial contraction dynamically by systolic extension. The interlaminar shear contributed about 40% and the extension component about 60% to ventricular transmural thickening. The ventricular thickening increased to almost 50% for only 13% myocyte shortening so that myocyte deformation from strain relative to fiber orientation influenced these findings. It has been estimated that systolic wall thickening could account for 25–50% of stroke volume.

More detailed knowledge of myocardial fiber structure, particularly the transmural gradient of fiber direction, and methods of measuring local deformation at different sites across the wall allows us to inquire about the relation between local myocardial structure and local myocardial function and perhaps to gain insight into the mechanism of systolic wall thickening.

A focus of work on structure and function has been the relation between the local fiber orientation and the direction of the maximum shortening deformation [2]. A major finding was that the

V R. Parachuri, S.M. Adhyapak, *Ventricular Geometry in Post-Myocardial Infarction Aneurysms*,
DOI 10.1007/978-1-4471-2861-8_2, © Springer-Verlag London 2012

principal shortening direction and fiber direction were almost parallel in the outer wall but perpendicular in the inner wall, where shortening was greatest near the circumferential direction; this shortening was accompanied by substantial wall thickening. It was concluded that some form of geometric rearrangement of myocytes was necessary for this deformation to occur. Wall thinning during passive filling at increasing pressures in rat hearts was associated with a reorientation of layers of myocytes, which apparently slid along transmurally oriented cleavage planes between the layers. One mode of deformation during systole may be a movement of the endocardium downward relative to the inner wall regions, giving rise to a positive shearing deformation (relative upward movement of the endocardium would be a negative shearing deformation). If we also assume that the myocardial laminae are stiff relative to the shearing stiffness of the space between them (not unreasonable in systole), then they will tend to slide relative to one another, causing the endocardial surface to displace into the LV cavity as it moves down in systole, contributing to local wall thickening. This mechanism of systolic wall thickening is supplemented to a small degree by increases in myocyte diameter as they shorten along their axis. In fact, significant positive shear in the LV free wall has been a consistent observation in studies of regional mechanics in normal myocardium.

Furthermore, in studies of regional mechanics in acutely ischemic myocardium, significant systolic wall thickening changed to thinning, and this was accompanied by a marked reduction or reversal of shear. These results further support the idea that there is a direct link between systolic wall thickening and transmural shearing deformation. The laminar myocardial structure with sheets of myocytes separated by cleavage planes seems to be designed for such a deformation. One might expect that the maximum relative sliding occurring in the myocardium is therefore coplanar with the myocardial sheets. Toward the endocardium, the shearing forces and myocardial laminae come into alignment such that there is maximum relative sliding between myocardial laminae, producing significant wall thickening [3].

The various axes of ventricular wall displacement are considered below.

Radial displacement: This is directed inward throughout the LV. The magnitude is greatest in the apical inferior and lateral walls and least in the septum and apicoanterior wall, reflecting contraction and bulk rotation about a septolateral axis with anterior motion at the apex. Shortening strains are maximal at the apex, moving axially from apex to base, causing descent of the mitral annulus.

Longitudinal deformation: Shortening along the long axis occurs by descent of the base toward the apex. The displacement magnitudes are greatest at the base, decreasing linearly toward the apex.

Circumferential deformation: When viewed from the base, it is clockwise initially, and anticlockwise up to end systole. More apically, the initial rotation is more prominent [4–5]. The magnitude of circumferential deformation is maximal at the base of the ventricle at its posterolateral walls. It is lesser in the anterior and anterolateral walls. But, it was greater than longitudinal shortening in the anterior wall but not in the posterior wall. The maximal stretch is associated with maximal wall thickening, and circumferential shortening is associated with maximal contraction.

Torsion: Torsion is the rotation of a level about the long axis with respect to the base. It is greater in the endocardium than the epicardium [4]. It is a function of the oblique ventricular fibers. In systole, the apex has a brief initial clockwise twist (torsion) followed by a predominant anticlockwise twist. The base twists in a clockwise direction (reverse of apical twist) causing a wringing effect enhancing ventricular ejection. In diastole, LV torsion occurs in the reverse direction – both the apex and the base twist in reverse of the systolic twist. This untwisting is maximal during early relaxation and augments LV filling by a suction effect [5]. The orientation of the oblique myocardial fibers is decisive of ventricular shape and function (Fig. 2.1).

The fiber angle is crucial for fiber obliquity. The normal oblique fiber angle is 60°. When heart failure ensues, the fiber orientation changes

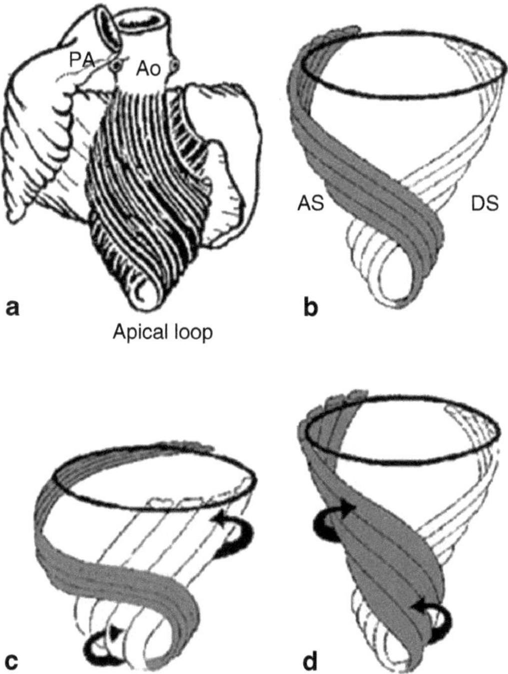

Fig. 2.1 Proposed role of sequential contraction of the ascendent and descendent segments of the ventricular band in the ejection and suction of blood. (**a**) The basal loop has been removed to expose the apical loop, pulmonary artery (*PA*), aorta (*Ao*) (**b**) formed by the descendent (*DS*) and ascendent (*AS*) segments; (**c**) during systole, the base of the heart is pulled downward, toward the apex, due to the contraction of the descendent segment (*thick bundles*). This results in shortening of the left ventricular cavity and results in ventricular ejection. Such a movement of the DS forces the ascendent segment to adopt a curvilinear configuration. Subsequent contraction (*thick bundles*) (**d**) uncoils and undoes the configurational change and allows sudden upward movement of the base of the heart, resulting in expansion of ventricular cavity and ventricular filling. The torsion and untorsion motion of the ventricles extensively described in magnetic resonance studies can be explained by the angled spatial distribution of the descendent and ascendent and fibers. (With permission from Roscitano et al. [7] Copyright Elsevier)

from oblique to transverse as detailed below. Sallin and coworkers [6] demonstrated that a myofiber contraction of 15% in a ventricle with a normal short/long axis ratio with a sphericity index of 0.5 (ellipsoid ventricular shape) generated an ejection fraction of 62%. At the same 15% fiber contraction, the ejection fraction fell below 40% if the sphericity index approached 1 (spherical ventricular shape) and went up to ≥80% if the sphericity index approached 0 (extreme ellipsoid ventricular shape).

Despite different torsions from base to apex and between epicardium and endocardium, these areas are subject to a constant mean shear. There is a circumferential-longitudinal shear – shear $_{CL}$ – at both epicardium and endocardium. It is constant from base to apex and from epicardium to endocardium.

Shear at a point is dependent on the torsion angle, the distance between the point and the center of the ventricular cavity (r), and the distance between the point and the base (h) (Fig. 2.2). The torsion increases as h increases and as r decreases. The torsion angle is maximal at the apex. The mean torsion angle of the endocardium is greater than that of the epicardium by approximately twofold. The nonlinear increase in torsion, with greater increments at the apex than at the base, is due to tapering at the apex [8]. The constancy of mean shear is maintained by variation in the torsion angle between apex to base and across the ventricular wall [4–6, 8–13]. This is the principle by which stress is equalized along the spatially nonhomogenous LV wall during normal ejection. The torsion of the epicardial fibers exceed that of the endocardial fibers [1, 4], as they are at a greater radius from the LV central long axis and so have longer lever arms to produce greater momentum. Also, torsion in the posteroseptal regions was less than in the anterolateral regions.

The normal right ventricular free wall also exhibits torsion, but of a lesser magnitude [9]. In patients who underwent Mustard or Senning repair for transposition of great arteries, the systemic right ventricle exhibited greater circumferential than longitudinal strain, in contrast to the normal right ventricle which has greater longitudinal than circumferential strain. This could be an adaptation to a higher resistance circulation. However, the systemic right ventricle did not exhibit any torsional movement. Torsion is a prerequisite for energy efficient LV ejection and relaxation. This is explained by the double helical myofiber structure and the acute angle between the LV inflow and outflow. This is impaired in myocardial

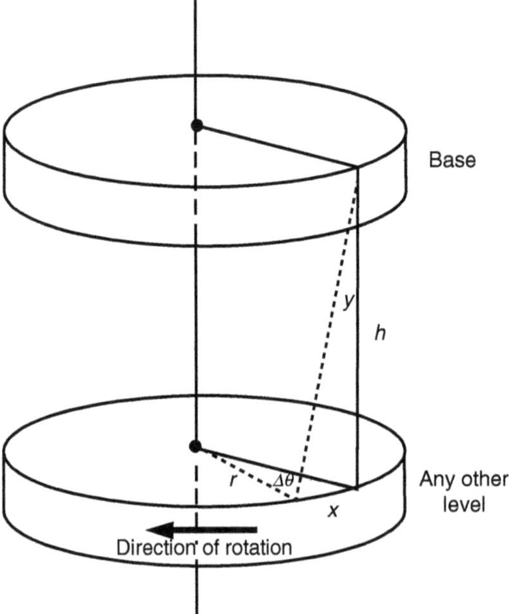

Fig. 2.2 Diagram illustrating torsion angle (θ) and shear$_{CL}$(γ) for one tag point. r is radius of epicardium, x is displacement of tag point, and h is distance between basal plane and succeeding plane (With permission from Buchalter et al. [4] Copyright LWW journals)

infarction, cardiomyopathy, and aortic stenosis and is more marked for diastolic untwisting, forming the basis of diastolic dysfunction in these disease states [10–12].

Physiological Variables Affecting Left Ventricular Twist

The left ventricular twist increases gradually from infancy to adulthood. Counterclockwise apical rotation is constant in magnitude in childhood, whereas the basal rotation changes over age, initially counterclockwise in infancy to neutral in early childhood to the adult clockwise pattern in adolescence [14]. This progressive change has been attributed to the maturation of the helical myofiber architecture of the left ventricular wall. Subsequently, with increasing age, subendocardial function gradually attenuates, and left ventricular twist increases further due to an unopposed increase in left ventricular apical rotation. Age-related degenerative changes reduce elastic resilience of the myocardial wall, and therefore velocity of untwisting in early diastole progressively reduces.

Physiological variables such as preload, afterload, and contractility alter the magnitude of left ventricular twist. The twist is greater with higher preload. For example, with higher left ventricular end diastolic volumes, with end systolic volume held constant, the left ventricular twist increases. Similarly, afterload affects twist, that is, twist decreases at higher end systolic volumes when end diastolic volumes are held constant. The effect of reload on twist is about two-thirds as great as that of afterload. Increasing contractility increases twist.

In the intact circulation, changes in contractility are often accompanied by changes in loading conditions for increasing the twist mechanics of the left ventricle. For example, systolic twisting and untwisting can almost double with short-term exercise due to augmented rotation of both apical and basal levels, storing additional potential energy that is released for improving diastolic suction. Long-term exercise training may however reduce twist at rest. Soccer players show lower twist values and untwisting velocities than nontrained individuals. It has been postulated that reduced twist in soccer players may represent increased torsional reserves that are used in increased demand situations such as high-intensity sports. The higher resting twist value seen with advancing age is associated with attenuation of torsional reserves at peak exercise.

Clinical Applications

Diastolic Dysfunction

Assessment of twist and peak untwisting rates were proposed to accurately reflect left ventricular relaxation. The left ventricular twist may be preserved in patients with diastolic dysfunction and normal ejection fraction. The twisting and untwisting rates were reduced in patients with systolic dysfunction and depressed ejection fraction. The onset of untwisting was significantly delayed after aortic valve closure in patients with systolic and diastolic heart failure. In hypertension, early diastolic untwisting and untwisting rates were significantly delayed and reduced in parallel to the severity of left ventricular hypertrophy.

Myocardial Ischemia and Infarction

In patients with anterior wall myocardial infarction, peak circumferential strain in the apex is significantly depressed in those patients with systolic dysfunction as compared with those with preserved systolic function. The twist is severely depressed in presence of systolic dysfunction mainly due to reduced magnitude of apical rotation. The diastolic untwisting is also reduced and delayed. In those patients with preserved systolic function, there is marginal reduction of apical circumferential strain and preservation of the apical twist. In patients with predominant subendocardial ischemia, there was greater than normal apical rotation, as rotation reflects subepicardial function which was preserved in these patients. With transmural ischemia, there was less than normal apical rotation.

The Mechanics of the Normal Cardiac Cycle

The functional mechanical patterns include an initial global counterclockwise twist (as seen from the apex) and attendant narrowing in the isovolumetric contraction phase. This is followed by continuing counterclockwise twisting of the apex and clockwise twisting of the base, as the ventricle longitudinally shortens during the ejection phase [15–18]. This is followed by a vigorous apical untwisting in the opposite direction as the ventricle lengthens and slightly widens during the isovolumetric relaxation phase when no blood enters or leaves the ventricle (Fig. 2.3). This is associated with a rapid ventricular pressure decay (tau) – a quantifiable rate of untwisting, followed by the rapid filling phase when suction occurs together with a recordable intraventricular pressure gradient, until a phase of relaxation occurs during diastole when ventricular widening continues by slower filling. This is followed by atrial contraction and the next beat ensues.

Regional Nonuniformity of Shape and Wall Movement in the Normal Left Ventricle

The shape of the left ventricle is nonhomogenous. The apex has the greatest curvature, while the posterior wall has a negative end diastolic curvature which decreases further at early systole and becomes positive at end systole. The anterior region has greatest, and the anteroapical region has the least fractional shortening. Asynchrony is evident as a delayed contraction of inferoapical and anteroapical regions with a greater rate of late systolic shortening of the anterior wall than that of the apex. Shape changes and shortening were dyssynchronous in the apical regions where the greatest changes occur in early diastole, which merits further study [20].

Regional Ejection Fraction in the Left Ventricle

There are differences in regional ejection fraction around the left ventricular circumference. The regions with the highest ejection fraction show least wall thickening, in the posterior and lateral walls. The regions with lower ejection fraction show greater wall thickening, in the anterior wall and septum. Conversely, a higher ejection fraction coincides with a larger epicardial inward motion (posterior epicardial circumferential shortening is twice that of anteroseptal region). This relationship between ejection fraction and thickening is not constant throughout the left ventricle. This can be explained by two factors, both related to left ventricular architecture. Wall thickness and radius of curvature are important determinants of wall stress. A more curved wall will exhibit less wall stress, leading to a thinner wall at end diastole, which will show a relative larger thickening for the same amount of increase in wall thickness. On the other hand, a smaller systolic stress will

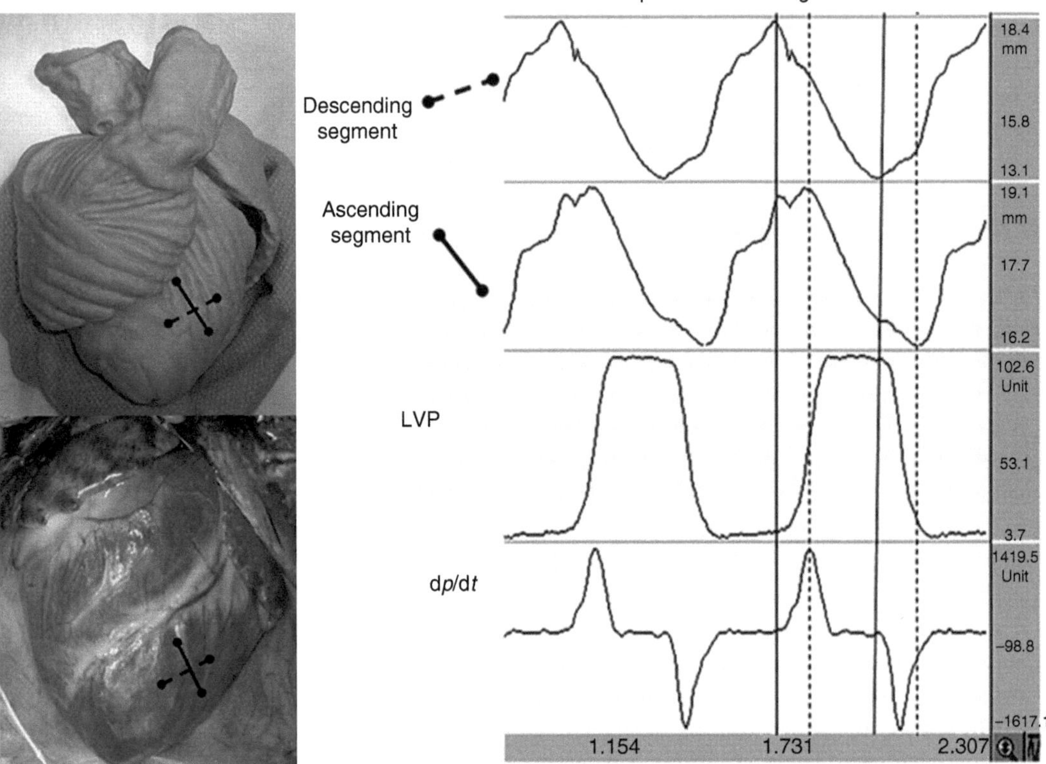

Fig. 2.3 Sonomicrometer crystal recording of systolic shortening in the descending (endocardial) and ascending (epicardial) fibers of the apical loop of the myocardial band. Crystals record maximal shortening when placed in this angulation of muscle fibers, and these tracings show shortening of the endocardial muscle during the interval that no motion is observed by radionuclide ventriculography (With permission from Bernal et al. [19] Copyright Elsevier)

allow a larger systolic regional ejection fraction. The balance between these two effects determines the final relation between thickening and ejection fraction. This is in contrast to the relation between ejection fraction and circumferential endocardial shortening which is very tight in all these regions, and this also holds to a lesser degree for longitudinal shortening [21].

Structural and Functional Correlations of the Mechanical Sequence

Preejection Phase

At the onset of systole, the predominantly transverse circumferential muscle shortens along with the right-handed helix or descending segment to compress the central left- and right-handed helices like a stiff outer shell and causes the temporary longitudinal lengthening of the apex and base during preejection phase [22]. This phase is predominantly caused by the circumferential fiber contraction [23]. The consequence is rotation of the heart in a counterclockwise direction – the cocking motion. The radial shortening due to circumferential fiber contraction compresses the inner helix and causes bidirectional cavity lengthening [24]. The epicardial segment of the helix does not contract during this phase. This preejection stretch of the helix may "load" the muscles to produce a Starling effect for subsequent ejection [25, 26].

Ejection Phase

During ejection, the circumferential fibers continue to shorten along with the oblique fibers in the right- and left-handed helices which cocontract to shorten and thicken to empty the heart [27]. The circumferential fibers produce a horizontal counterforce that increases narrowing throughout ejection. They also provide a "buttress" to counteract the outer forces generated by the twisting and shortening oblique muscle fibers. The strain is greatest in the right-handed endocardial helix and is responsible for shortening and clockwise twisting of the cardiac base. The simultaneous counterclockwise apical twist is due to torsion of the left-handed epicardial helix with a larger radius of curvature [28]. This interaction is responsible for systolic torsion.

A network of connected fibers exist between transverse and oblique fibers which induces shear by creating transmural torsion [29]. As the right-handed helix contraction dominates to shorten the ventricular chamber, it pulls down the left-handed helix whose fibers become horizontally oriented. This helical cocontraction joins circumferential contraction to increase chamber narrowing during ejection to facilitate propulsion of blood [6]. Deformation is greatest toward the apex, to achieve maximal reduction in chamber volume which is explained by the anatomical fact that the right- and left-handed helices converge toward the apex to form the vortex of the double helical loop [21, 30]. Each spiral arm of the helix globally twists itself in opposite directions, the right-handed helix being dominant, and is directed downward, and its twist causes the observed clockwise rotation of the cardiac base. The left-handed helix twists counterclockwise to produce apical reciprocal rotation. Although the apical longitudinal motion is directed upward, it predominantly moves downward as it is dominated by the right-handed helix. The entire left-handed helix twists counterclockwise at the apex and appears as a leftward direction of the upper septum that correlates movement with the anatomic wrap around configuration. Simultaneously, it thickens to compress the cavity, but its effort to elevate the ventricle is offset by the prevailing dominance of the right-handed helix. This contraction-related elevation of the left-handed helix only becomes apparent during the isovolumetric contraction phase when the right-handed helix contraction stops. From a mechanical point, the shortening motion during ejection reflects the dominant force of the right-handed helix than the constrictive motion of the circumferential fibers which predominantly cause compression.

Isovolumetric Relaxation Phase

After ejection, the right-handed helix stops contracting but maintains stiffness and tension and thus acts as a fulcrum for the left-handed helix straightening as this segment continues to contract in an unopposed fashion for an additional 90 ms [31]. When a helix is compressed, its two ends approach each other, and the internal coils become more horizontal [31, 32]. When stretched, the two ends move apart and the coils become more vertical and the helix becomes straighter. Cavity widening occurs without blood inflow and is related to the recoil of the circumferential muscle that has stopped contracting. The predominant motion is rapid clockwise untwisting of the apex and midwall, together with increased clockwise motion of the base. These movements occur before the end of systole and exist only when the left-handed helix is contracting. The widening of the base is associated with lengthening of the base. The right-handed helix straightens as the left-handed helix maintains strain and continues to shorten.

The untwisting motion during elongation creates a negative pressure and potential vacuum that continues into the phase of rapid cavity filling after the decelerating ventricular pressure falls below atrial pressure [33]. Its origin is likely from titin-related recoil of the noncontracting circumferential fibers that exerted a counterclockwise rotation during preejection [32]. The right-handed helix straightens as the left-handed helix maintains strain and continues to shorten and elevates. So, the left-handed helix cannot be the cause of untwisting. The clockwise rotation of the apex is governed by recoil of the circumferential fibers which stop contracting and is the opposite movement from the preejection counterclockwise motion. Although the apex continues its counterclockwise motion because of the left-handed helix, its radial velocity forces are markedly diminished. Therefore, the observed net clockwise motion reflects untwisting of the apex from recoil of the circumferential fibers.

Conversely, an opposite action exists for the circumferential muscle in preparation for ventricular filling, as untwisting and widening develop a potential intraventricular vacuum for subsequent suction during unopposed straightening of the left-handed helix [34, 35]. The cardiac base widens and the chamber cavity lengthens while maintaining its thickness [33]. The circumferential muscle exerts a balancing action by preventing explosion during filling and ejection. The oblique fibers govern the shortening and lengthening motions.

Rapid Filling Phase

The suction phase for rapid filling occurs after ventricular pressure falls below atrial pressure and is associated with a further rapid accentuation of untwisting of the apex in a clockwise direction. It has been shown that 40% of untwisting occurs before the rapid filling phase [36]. The continued untwisting is caused by elastic recoil of compressed titin coils within the left-handed helix fibers, in a manner similar to circumferential muscle widening and recoil for clockwise rotation during the isovolumic phase [37]. As the contractile phase dissipates, and all muscle segments become relaxed, the rapid titin-related unwinding of the apex to its original position creates the suction required for rapid ventricular filling, which occurs as the ventricular pressure drops below the atrial pressure [38]. Further widening and lengthening develop from the hydraulic effects resulting from rapid and then passive filling after apical reciprocal twisting has stopped.

Further investigations of these spatial anatomic and physiological concepts are needed to allow accurate understanding of the mechanisms of cardiac dynamics.

References

1. Moore CC, McVeigh ER, Elias A. Quantitative tagged magnetic resonance imaging of the normal human ventricle. Top Magn Reson Imaging. 2000;11(6): 359–71.
2. Osakada G, Sasayama S, Kawai C, Hirakawa A, Kemper WS, Franklin D, Ross Jr J. The analysis of left ventricular wall thickness and shear by an ultrasonic triangulation technique in the dog. Circ Res. 1980;47: 173–81.
3. LeGrice IJ, Takayama Y, Covell JW. Transverse shear along myocardial cleavage planes provides a mechanism for normal systolic wall thickening. Circ Res. 1995;77:182–93.
4. Buchalter MB, Weiss JL, Rogers WJ, Zerhouni EA, Weissfeldt ML, Beyar R, Shapiro EP. Noninvasive quantification of left ventricular rotational deformation in normal humans using MRI myocardial tagging. Circulation. 1990;81:1236–44.
5. Ashikaga H, Criscione JC, Omens JH, Covell JW, Ingels NB. Transmural left ventricular mechanics underlying torsional recoil during relaxation. Am J Physiol Heart Circ Physiol. 2004;286:H640–7.
6. Sallin EA. Fiber orientation and ejection fraction in the human ventricle. Biophys J. 1969;9:954–64.
7. Roscitano A, Benedetto U, Sciangula A, Merico E, Barberi F, Bianchini R, Tonelli E, Sinatra R. Indexed effective orifice area after mechanical aortic valve replacement does not affect left ventricular mass regression in elderly. Eur J Cardiothorac Surg. 2006;29: S139–43.
8. Badeer HS. Contractile tension in the myocardium. Am Heart J. 1963;66:432–7.
9. Pettersen E, Vale TH, Lindberg EH, Smith HJ, Smevik B, Andersen K. Contraction pattern of the systemic right ventricle. J Am Coll Cardiol. 2007;49:2450–6.
10. Nagel E, Stuber M, Lakatos M, Scheidegger MB, Boesiger P, Hess OM. Cardiac rotation and relaxation after anterolateral myocardial infarction. Coron Artery Dis. 2000;11:261–7.
11. Stuber M, Scheidegger MB, Fischer SC, Nagel E, Steinmann F, Hess OM, Boesiger P. Alterations in the local myocardial motion pattern in patients suffering from pressure overload due to aortic stenosis. Circulation. 1999;100:361–8.
12. Tibiyan FA, Lai DT, Timek TA, Dagum P, Liang D, Daughters GT, Ingels NB, Miller DC. Alterations in left ventricular torsion in tachycardia induced dilated cardiomyopathy. J Thorac Cardiovasc Surg. 2002;124: 43–9.
13. Sandler H, Dodge HT. Left ventricular tension and stress in man. Circ Res. 1963;13:91–104.
14. Sengupta P, Tajik J, Krishnaswamy C, Khanderia BK. Twist mechanics of the left ventricle. JACC Cardiovasc Imaging. 2008;1:366–76.
15. Young AA, Imai H, Chang CN, Axel L. Two-dimensional left ventricular deformation during systole using MRI with spatial modulation of magnetization. Circulation. 1994;89:740–52.
16. Axel L, Gonsalves R, Bloomgarden D. Regional heart wall motion: two-dimensional analysis and functional imaging of regional heart wall motion with MRI. Radiology. 1992;183:745–50.
17. Rogers W, Shapiro E, Weiss J. Quantification of and correction for left ventricular systolic long-axis

shortening by MR tissue tagging and slice isolation. Circulation. 1991;84:721–31.
18. Reichek N. MRI for assessment of myocardial function. Magn Reson Q. 1991;7:255–74.
19. Bernal JM, Lorca J, Prieto-Salceda D, Pulitani I, Pontón A, García I, Revuelta JM. Performance at 10 years of the CarboMedics 'Top Hat' valve. Postclamping time is a predictor of mortality. Eur J Cardiothorac Surg. 2006;29:S144–9.
20. Barletta G, Baroni M, Del Bene R, Toso A, Fantini F. Regional and temporal non uniformity of shape and wall movement in the normal left ventricle. Cardiology. 1998;90:195–201.
21. Bogaert J, Rademakers FE. Regional nonuniformity of normal adult human left ventricle. Am J Physiol. 2001;280:H610–20.
22. Buckberg G, Hoffman J, Mahajan A, Saleh S, Coghlan C. Cardiac mechanics revisited: the relationship of cardiac architecture to ventricular function. Circulation. 2008;118:2571–87.
23. McDonald IG. The shape and movements of the human left ventricle during systole: a study by cineangiography and by cineradiography of epicardial markers. Am J Cardiol. 1970;26:221–30.
24. Sengupta PP, Khandheria BK, Korinek J, Jahangir A, Yoshifuku S, Milosevic I, Belohlavek M. Left ventricular isovolumic flow sequence during sinus and paced rhythms: new insights from use of high-resolution Doppler and ultrasonic digital particle imaging velocimetry. J Am Coll Cardiol. 2007;49:899–908.
25. Buckberg GD, Castella M, Gharib M, Saleh S. Structure/function interface with sequential shortening of basal and apical components of the myocardial band. Eur J Cardiothorac Surg. 2006;29 Suppl 1:S75–97.
26. Sengupta PP, Korinek J, Belohlavek M, Narula J, Vannan MA, Jahangir A, Khandheria BK. Left ventricular structure and function: basic science for cardiac imaging. J Am Coll Cardiol. 2006;48:1988–2001.
27. Sengupta PP, Krishnamorthy VK, Korinek J, Narula J, Vannan MA, Lester SJ, Tajik JA, Seward JB, Khandheria BK, Belohlavek M. Left ventricular form and function revisited: applied translational science to cardiovascular ultrasound imaging. J Am Soc Echocardiogr. 2007;20:539–51.
28. Thomas JD, Popovic ZB. Assessment of left ventricular function by cardiac ultrasound. J Am Coll Cardiol. 2006;48:2012–25.
29. Anderson RH, Siew YH, Sanchez-Quintana D, Redmann K, Lunkenheimer PP. Heuristic problems in defining the three-dimensional arrangement of the ventricular myocytes. Anat Rec. 2006;288A:579–86.
30. Ingels NB, Hansen D, Daughters II GT, Stinson EB, Alderman E, Miller DC. Relation between longitudinal, circumferential, and oblique shortening and torsional deformation in the left ventricle of the transplanted human heart. Circ Res. 1989;64:915–27.
31. Jung B, Markl M, Foll D, Buckberg GD, Hennig J. Investigating myocardial motion by MRI using tissue phase mapping. Eur J Cardiothorac Surg. 2006;29 Suppl 1:S150–7.
32. Katz AM, Zile MR. New molecular mechanism in diastolic heart failure. Circulation. 2006;113:1922–5.
33. Nikolic SD, Feneley MP, Pajaro OE, Rankin JS, Yellin EL. Origin of regional pressure gradients in the left ventricle during early diastole. Am J Physiol. 1995;268:H550–7.
34. Davis KL, Mehlhorn U, Schertel ER, Geissler HJ, Trevas D, Laine GA, Allen SJ. Variation in tau, the time constant for isovolumic relaxation, along the left ventricular base-to-apex axis. Basic Res Cardiol. 1999;94:41–8.
35. Simari RD, Bell MR, Schwartz RS, Nishimura RA, Holmes Jr DR. Ventricular relaxation and myocardial ischemia: a comparison of different models of tau during coronary angioplasty. Cathet Cardiovasc Diagn. 1992;25:278–84.
36. Dong SJ, Hees PS, Siu CO, Weiss JL, Shapiro EP. MRI assessment of LV relaxation by untwisting rate: a new isovolumic phase measure of tau. Am J Physiol. 2001;281:H2002–9.
37. Stuber M, Scheidegger MB, Fischer SE, Nagel E, Steinemann F, Hess OM. Alterations in the local myocardial motion pattern in patients suffering from pressure overload due to aortic stenosis. Circulation. 1999;100:361–8.
38. Castella M, Buckberg GD. Diastolic dysfunction in stunned myocardium and its prevention by Na+-H+exchange inhibition. Eur J Cardiothorac Surg. 2006;29 Suppl 1:S107–14.

Altered Left Ventricular Geometry in Ischemic Cardiomyopathy

3

Introduction

With the advent of heart failure, significant changes imprint its underlying pathology and distort the normal left ventricular architecture leading to perturbations in ventricular function. The early changes of increased spherical configuration lead to impairment of ventricular function during exercise and may lead to exercise-induced functional mitral regurgitation. With advanced heart failure, extensive ventricular remodeling occurs when only pharmacological therapy may not suffice. Therapy in these scenarios will require an extensive armamentarium of devices and nontransplant surgeries. This chapter deals with the perturbations in cardiac anatomy following transmural myocardial infarctions and aneurysm formation. The intrinsic myofiber orientations are distorted with ventricular wall thinning and fibrosis, replacing portions of the ventricular wall. The cellular mechanisms involved in the remodeling process have also been detailed.

In chronic heart failure, there is dilatation of the cardiac chambers, which leads to distortion of the LV ellipsoid geometry [1]. At the base, dilatation leads to straightening of the angle between the LV inflow and outflow. The oblique fibers from mid-wall to apex become more horizontal [1–3]. A theoretical analysis can demonstrate that an oblique fiber angle on a surface with a certain radius of curvature (Fig. 3.1) can attain a narrower angle, as the surface projects onto one with a larger radius of curvature as in a dilated spherical ventricle. For example, for a normal 60° fiber angle, increase in short axis dimension of the ellipsoid by 3 cm can decrease the fiber angle by 10° that is from 60° to 50°. Minor fiber angle changes of 5°–10° can substantially affect ventricular torsion and performance [5].

If the left ventricle dilates because of myocardial injury, the following associated changes occur. Ventricular shape becomes more spherical, making the circumferential shortening and wall thickening markedly decrease. The myocardial fiber orientation changes as detailed above, and meridional stress increases, while equatorial stress remains within normal limits.

However, if the ventricle dilates uniformly due to volume overload with intact myocardial function as in valvular regurgitations, the ventricular shape, circumferential shortening, wall thickening, and fiber orientation remain relatively intact compared with damaged hearts of equivalent size; both meridional- and equatorial-calculated wall stresses increase, and to the same degree, but the changes may not reflect increased force per myocardial fiber if shape and fiber orientation are taken into consideration [6]. This clearly demonstrates that fiber orientation affects shape which ultimately affects ventricular function profoundly.

Ventricular remodeling is a progressive process, which starts very soon after a myocardial infarction, even though its clinical symptoms may not be demonstrated for years. A consensus statement defined remodeling as "the genomic expression resulting in molecular, cellular, and

V R. Parachuri, S.M. Adhyapak, *Ventricular Geometry in Post-Myocardial Infarction Aneurysms*,
DOI 10.1007/978-1-4471-2861-8_3, © Springer-Verlag London 2012

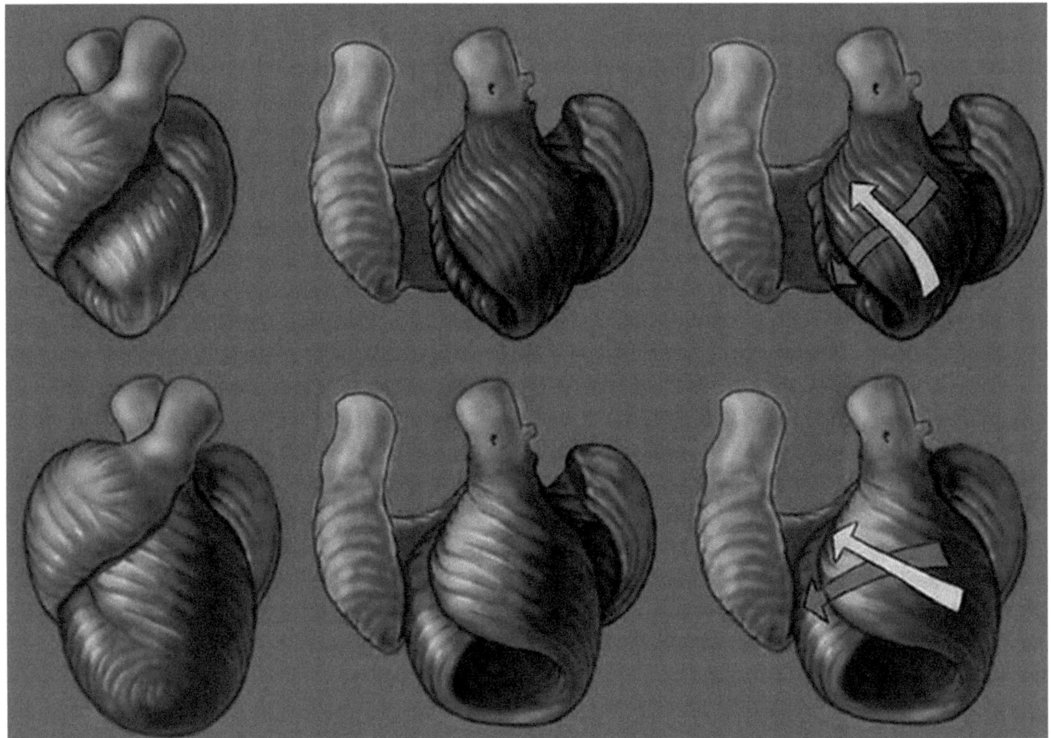

Fig. 3.1 Comparison of the normal and dilated heart, whereby the architectural patterns of the apical loop change from an oblique orientation to a more transverse pattern and begin to resemble the horizontal basal loop configuration (With permission from Coghlan and Hoffman [4] Copyright Elsevier)

interstitial changes that are manifested clinically as changes in size, shape, and function of the heart after cardiac injury" [7]. Most of our understanding of ventricular remodeling stems from studies performed on patients after myocardial infarctions, although remodeling can occur after any type of cardiac injury, like myocarditis, hypertension, or valvular disease.

Remodeling has fundamentally been described by the anatomic changes in the left ventricle after an infarction, both within the infarcted and non-infarcted myocardium. After an epicardial coronary artery occludes, the underperfused myocardium develops ischemia and infarcts. In infarcted myocardium, both the myocytes and intercellular components are affected. In the first day post-infarction, the myocytes undergo necrosis and the collagen fibers, which hold the muscle cells in place, begin to degrade in quality and number [8]. Around post-infarction days, three to four, the inflammatory cells, such as macrophages, infiltrate the necrotic tissue [9, 10]. Soon after this, at day 4 or 5, the infarction begins to expand [9]. Infarction expansion, as described by Hutchins and Buckley [9], involves an acute dilatation and wall thinning of the infarcted area without additional necrosis, which leads to left ventricular cavity dilation. Within the infarcted myocardium, multiple mechanisms likely contribute to wall thinning, including cell stretching (an increase in sarcomere length) and a reduction in intercellular space, such as the capillary beds, which together increase the cell density in the infarct area [10]; however, wall thinning occurs primarily by a sliding movement of the myocytes by a mechanism termed "slippage" [10]. In the predominant method of wall thinning in the infarcted tissue, slippage happens mainly because, by post-infarction day 4, the collagen and collagen struts [8], which hold the collagen to myocytes, have degraded sufficiently through necrosis permitting the cellular movement. Infarct expansion occurs before the necrosis resorption by macrophages and other inflammatory cells [9]. The infarcted left ventricle dilates regionally during this expansion. As the infarction is expanding, cardiac fibroblasts deposit collagen on the already thinned tissue. Once enough collagen accumulates, a scar forms which resists further expansion [8].

Outside of the infarction, the non-infarcted left ventricle continues to remodel over the proceeding weeks to months. Most importantly, the non-infarcted cardiomyocytes develop eccentric hypertrophy, an end-to-end, lengthwise growth, similar to a volume-overload hypertrophy [11], that results in left ventricular cavity dilation. The non-infarcted myocardium undergoes wall thinning with cardiomyocytes sliding side by side, "slippage," by loss of intercellular connections [10, 12]. Initially, the compensatory hypertrophy in the remote myocardium is beneficial because it compensates for the functional loss of the infarcted myocardium. However, over time, this adaptive hypertrophy becomes detrimental because the increased ventricular radius increases the wall stress by Laplace law and thus increases oxygen demand [11]. Hemodynamic changes within the post-infarcted left ventricle occur in association with these anatomical adaptations: as the ventricular chamber dilates with increased end-diastolic and end-systolic volumes, the left ventricular filling pressure/pulmonary capillary wedge pressure initially decrease in the post-infarction ventricle [13]. At first, these adaptations appear beneficial; however, as the ventricle continues to dilate, the wall stress increases in the infarcted ventricle. As the myocardium continues to develop eccentric hypertrophy and wall thinning, the left ventricular volume (LV cavity size) increases at a rate faster than the myocardial mass. This mismatch between left ventricular volume and wall thickness results in increased wall stress, with decreased subendocardial perfusion and, ultimately, in depressed LV ejection fraction [14].

The adverse left ventricular remodeling has been described following transmural myocardial infarctions [15]. The fibrotic scar formation has been demonstrated by MRI as being located along the midmyocardium, rather than the endomyocardium or epimyocardium [16].

Early after myocardial infarctions, that is, 1 week following infarction, the wall thickening is relatively unaffected. This can be explained by the laminar myocardial fiber architecture. The systolic slippage of laminar sheets in the myocardium is a critical factor for generating wall thickness. Even if the mid-circumferential myofibers are dysfunctional or injured, slippage of the laminar sheet may generate enough of a longitudinal gap between the epi- and endomyocardial surfaces during an infarction or immediately after, if the width of the laminar sheet is kept normal and the rest of the myocardium is functional [16].

The border and remote zones demonstrate a decrease in wall thickening 4 weeks following myocardial infarctions. Myocardial scar extension also occurs along the midmyocardium. This scar extension is a critical predictor of adverse left ventricular remodeling in the chronic phase [16], which leads to left ventricular aneurysm formation.

Ventricular Remodeling After an Anterior Wall Myocardial Infarction

It is well known that anteroapical MIs have a greater influence on LV function than do "similarly sized infarctions" in other regions of the LV [17]. This is likely related to morphologic changes in the infarct-related myocardium, influencing the behavior of the remote myocardium. The following paragraph may give a new view on the mechanism of remote myocardial dysfunction in patients with an anterior MI.

First, LV ejection is partially caused by longitudinal LV shortening, which mainly relies on the obliquely oriented endocardial and epicardial fibers. Impaired longitudinal shortening in the remote myocardium very likely relies on increased longitudinal wall stress secondary to morphologic changes in the infarct-related myocardium or to changes in LV shape and may represent a kind of longitudinal tethering. As shown here, wall expansion in the infarct area increases the longitudinal radius of curvature in the apex and exposes this wall segment to greater intramural tension. Subsequently, the longitudinal wall stress will increase in the remote areas and will lead to wall flattening (as shown by the increase in the longitudinal radius of curvature). This effect is more pronounced endocardially than epicardially, leading to greater endocardial longitudinal wall stress and a reversal of the longitudinal–radial shear strain. The importance of a normal longitudinal–radial shear strain in providing normal myocardial function has been stressed. Although wall stress has not mathematically calculated, directional changes can be deduced reliably from alterations in the determinants of wall stress (i.e., radius of curvature).

Second, although the increase in the circumferential radius of curvature in the remote myocardium could act as a compensatory mechanism to improve LV function by increasing the regional preload, this compensatory mechanism seems to be ineffective because the circumferential shortening decreases in the remote myocardium. Circumferential shortening is more affected epicardially than endocardially. The latter can explain the preserved apparent systolic wall thickening in the remote myocardium while the centripetal systolic wall motion is significantly reduced, thus contributing to a reduction of regional EF in this part of the ventricle.

The specific morphologic changes are an increase in the regional radius of curvature of the expanded wall segment, an alteration in the spatial relation of the anterior and posterior papillary muscles, an increase in overall left ventricular diameter, and local wall thinning. Severe expansion has been associated with left ventricular aneurysm formation, as well as rupture of a myocardial infarct. Even in less severe cases, the increase in functional infarct size and of myocardial oxygen demands resulting from the morphologic alterations following expansion probably contribute further to cardiac dysfunction.

Role of Infarct Expansion in Ventricular Dilatation

The ventricle can expand within 48 h of a transmural infarction. It has been suggested that uninfarcted myocardial segments undergo diastolic lengthening by the Frank–Starling mechanism to compensate for the loss of contractile muscle mass. Studies in experimental infarct models show, however, that within minutes of acute ischemia, the infarct zone lengthens, as much or more than the uninfarcted muscle, possibly because of passive stretching of nonviable muscle segments during systole. In this study, we found that infarct expansion, as defined by an abnormally lengthened infarct segment, was the major contributor to ventricular dilation during the 72 h after infarction. Uninfarcted myocardial segments did not significantly contribute to acute left ventricular dilation. The lack of contribution of the uninfarcted segment to acute ventricular enlargement is to be contrasted with the situation at long-term follow-up in a study which showed general progressive ventricular dilation for more than 1 year, involving both the infarcted and uninfarcted segments. An abnormality in ventricular shape, characterized by an anteroseptal angulation, was seen. This abnormality was characterized by an abrupt angulation in the contour of the proximal anteroseptal wall in the long-axis echocardiographic view. Distal to the angulation, the wall is dyssynergic and bulges outward, increasing the size of the left ventricular cavity. Anteroseptal angulation was significantly associated with infarct expansion and was seen. Segmental dilation measured in the minor-axis view and anteroseptal angulation noted in the long-axis view may reflect the phenomenon of infarct expansion as viewed in two different planes. It has been shown that dilation of the left ventricle occurs within the first 24–72 h of anterior transmural myocardial infarction and is primarily due to lengthening of infarcted myocardial segments. Viable uninfarcted myocardial segments do not appear to participate significantly in the acute ventricular enlargement. By increasing the size of the left ventricle, infarct expansion causes an additional load to be placed on the remaining normal, functioning myocardium. Thus, infarcts of similar size with or without expansion may have differing effects on ventricular mechanics and clinical outcome.

Another consequence of infarct expansion is that the surface extent of infarcted myocardium is increased without any increase in infarct mass.

This bears importantly on methods of infarct size estimation that depend on measurement of the surface area of ventricular dysfunction or scintigraphic defect size. In the presence of infarct expansion, a method that measures the area but not the mass of abnormal myocardium is likely to overestimate the true infarct size in patients with infarct expansion [18].

Factors of Infarct Expansion Leading to Ventricular Aneurysm Formation

Moderate to marked infarct expansion was seen in almost half of all cases of myocardial infarctions and was highly correlated with the development of left ventricular aneurysm, as indicated by the degree of left ventricular contour break. A striking association between both the size of the myocardial infarct and the degree of transmurality of the myocardial infarct is indicated by the S/A thickness ratio (ratio of the thickness of surviving [S] muscle in the center of the infarct to the thickness of the adjacent [A] noninvolved myocardium) and the development of infarct expansion. The observation that infarct rupture was associated with a low S/A thickness ratio supports this concept. The degree of transmurality of the infarct influences the development of left ventricular aneurysm, with more transmural infarcts displaying a greater degree of aneurysmal change. It is possible that infarct expansion may be influenced by lesion location. This finding is supported by the striking tendency for myocardial infarcts in the distribution of the left anterior descending coronary artery to display moderate to marked degrees of expansion. This agrees with another study which found that anterior and anteroseptal myocardial infarcts were at high risk for expansion. Although infarcts in the distribution of the left anterior descending coronary artery were found to be significantly larger than infarcts in the distribution of either the left circumflex or right coronary artery, and thus at greater risk for expansion, multivariate regression analysis showed that infarct location in the distribution of the left anterior descending coronary artery was a distinct predictor of infarct expansion. Accordingly, regions of the left ventricular myocardium with the greatest radii of curvature experience the greatest intramural tension and, in response, thicken to the greatest degree. The effect of different radii of curvature on regional myocardial thickness is easily observed in the normal heart, where the apical myocardial wall has the smallest radius of curvature and is also noted to have the least cross-sectional wall thickness. One would therefore expect that those wall segments in the distribution of the left anterior descending coronary artery, which have relatively smaller radii of curvature (greatest degree of wall curvature), would be thinner than those myocardial segments in the distribution of the right coronary artery, which have relatively greater radii of curvature. These differences in the degree of normal segmental thickness may, in part, account for the increased tendency for infarct expansion observed between myocardial lesions in the distribution of the left anterior descending coronary artery and lesions in the distribution of the right coronary artery. In the normal left ventricle, the free wall in the distribution of the left circumflex coronary artery has the greatest thickness, while the free wall in the distribution of the left anterior descending coronary artery is thinnest. This differential thickness serves to promote differential degrees of transmurality of infarction, which in turn may be responsible for the different degrees of expansion observed in myocardial infarcts in different regions of the heart. Thus, severe infarction expansion is most often an event occurring in lesions in the distribution of the left anterior descending coronary artery, that is, in lesions that involve left ventricular wall segments that normally have the greatest degree of curvature [19].

Mechanics of Left Ventricular Aneurysm Formation

An acute infarct has very low stiffness, and if it involves the entire wall, there is a risk of rupture; however, in the absence of such a critical situation, fibrous tissue is laid into the infarcted myocardial segment. Such an infarcted fibrotic myocardial segment will not be able to contract, and so generate tensile stress. The surrounding intact myocardium will contract and generate wall stress, thereby developing a high intrachamber systolic pressure; the chronically infarcted and fibrotic segment will have to sustain this high chamber pressure. Its loss of contractility and the resulting reduced systolic stiffness relative to the intact segment will cause it to deform into a bulge; this is an aneurysm.

To determine the left ventricular wall deformation and the stress arising from infarction of a wall segment (which leads to a ventricular aneurysm), the left ventricle was modeled as a pressurized ellipsoidal shell. Deformations of infarcted wall segments were computed for several damaged wall thicknesses in left ventricles of different shapes. The analysis involved a derivation of equations for wall stress equilibrium with the chamber pressure and myocardial incompressibility before and after infarct formation.

The dependence of tensile stress and the bulge of infarcted wall segments on the extent of damaged wall thickness and the angle of infarct were computed.

The percentage of infarcted wall thickness and the shape of the ellipsoidal left ventricular chamber played more dominant roles than the angle of damage, or the extent of the infarct [20].

Definition of a Left Ventricular Aneurysm

Left ventricular aneurysm has been strictly defined as a distinct area of abnormal left ventricular diastolic contour with systolic dyskinesia or paradoxical bulging [15]. Yet a growing number of authors favor defining left ventricular aneurysm more loosely as any large area of left ventricular akinesia or dyskinesia that reduces left ventricular ejection fraction [21]. This broader definition has been justified by data suggesting that the pathophysiology and treatment may be the same for both ventricular akinesia and ventricular dyskinesia [22]. True left ventricular aneurysms involve bulging of the full thickness of the left ventricular wall.

Etiology of Left Ventricular Aneurysm

Over 95% of true left ventricular aneurysms reported in the English literature result from coronary artery disease and myocardial infarctions. True left ventricular aneurysms also may result from trauma, Chagas' disease [23], or sarcoidosis [24]. A very small number of congenital left ventricular aneurysms also have been reported and have been termed diverticula of the left ventricle [25].

Pathophysiology of Left Ventricular Aneurysm

The development of a true left ventricular aneurysm involves two principal phases: early expansion and late remodeling.

Early Expansion Phase

The early expansion phase begins with the onset of myocardial infarction. Ventriculography can demonstrate left ventricular aneurysm formation as early as within 48 h of infarction in 50% of patients who develop ventricular aneurysms. The remaining patients have evidence of aneurysm formation by 2 weeks after infarction [26].

True aneurysm of the left ventricle generally follows transmural myocardial infarction owing to acute occlusion of the left anterior descending artery (LAD) or dominant right coronary artery [27]. Lack of angiographic collaterals is strongly associated with aneurysm formation in patients with acute myocardial infarction (AMI) and LAD artery occlusion, and absence of re-formed collateral circulation is probably a prerequisite for the formation of a dyskinetic left ventricular aneurysm. At least 88% of dyskinetic ventricular aneurysms result from anterior infarction, whereas the remainder follow inferior infarction [28]. Posterior infarctions that produce a distinct dyskinetic left ventricular aneurysm are relatively unusual.

In experimental transmural infarction without collateral circulation, myocyte death begins 19 min after coronary occlusion. Infarctions that result in dyskinetic aneurysm formation are almost always transmural and may show gross thinning of the infarct zone within hours of infarction. Within a few days, the endocardial surface of the developing aneurysm becomes smooth with loss of trabeculae and deposition of fibrin and thrombus on the endocardial surface in at least 50% of patients. While most myocytes within the infarct are necrotic, viable myocytes often remain within the infarct zone. In a minority of patients, extravascular hemorrhage occurs in the infarcted tissue and may further depress systolic and diastolic function of involved myocardium. Inflammatory cells migrate into the infarct zone by 2–3 days after infarction and contribute to lysis of necrotic myocytes by 5–10 days after infarction. Electron microscopy demonstrates disruption of the native collagen network several days after infarction. Collagen disruption and myocyte necrosis produce a nadir of myocardial tensile strength between 5 and 10 days after infarction, when rupture of the myocardial wall is most common. Left ventricular rupture is relatively rare after the ventricular aneurysmal wall becomes replaced with fibrous tissue.

Loss of systolic contraction in the large infarcted zone and preserved contraction of surrounding myocardium cause systolic bulging and thinning of the infarct. By Laplace's law ($T=Pr/2h$), at a constant ventricular pressure P, increased radius of curvature r and decreased wall thickness h in the infarcted zone both contribute to increased muscle fiber tension T and further stretch the infarcted ventricular wall.

Relative to normal myocardium, ischemically, injured or infarcted myocardium displays greater plasticity or creep, defined as deformation or stretch over time under a constant load [29]. Thus, increased systolic and diastolic wall stress in the infarcted zone tends to produce progressive stretch of the infarcted myocardium (termed infarct expansion) until healing reduces the plasticity of the infarcted myocardium [30].

Left ventricular aneurysms can produce both systolic and diastolic ventricular dysfunction [31]. Diastolic dysfunction results from increased stiffness of the distended and fibrotic aneurysmal wall, which impairs diastolic filling and increases left ventricular end-diastolic (LVED) pressure.

Late Remodeling Phase

The remodeling phase of ventricular aneurysm formation begins 2–4 weeks after infarction when highly vascularized granulation tissue appears. This granulation tissue is replaced subsequently by fibrous tissue 6–8 weeks after infarction. As myocytes are lost, ventricular wall thickness decreases as the myocardium becomes largely replaced by fibrous tissue. In larger infarcts, the thin scar often is lined with mural thrombus [16, 21].

Lack of coronary reperfusion probably is a prerequisite for development of left ventricular aneurysm. In humans, reperfusion of the infarct vessel either spontaneously [32] by thrombolysis [33] or by angioplasty [34] has been associated with a lower incidence of aneurysm formation. It was speculated that coronary reperfusion as late as 2 weeks after infarction prevents aneurysm formation by improving blood flow and fibroblast migration into the infarcted myocardium, but aneurysms can still develop especially in large infarcts which can be predominantly akinetic instead of dyskinetic due to the presence of islands of viable myocardium within the scar.

At the Cellular Level: Replacement Fibrosis and Remodeling

Fibrosis, including microscopic scarring, is a fundamental component of the adverse structural remodeling found in the myocardium of the failing human heart [35, 36]. Scarring, a morphologic footprint of earlier cardiomyocyte necrosis, serves to replace lost contractile cells and thereby plays a vital role in preserving myocardial structure and function. The extensive distribution of this replacement fibrosis suggests a widespread and ongoing necrosis of cardiomyocytes. Apoptosis also occurs in the failing heart, but to a lesser extent, often involving such noncardiomyocytes as macrophages and endothelial cells [37]. Furthermore, programmed cell death begets neither inflammatory cells nor fibroblast responses. As a consequence, fibrous tissue does not appear at the site of lost myocytes and, therefore, apoptosis has been referred to as a sterile form of cell death [38, 39]. The cumulative loss of contractile elements, together with the deposition of fibrous tissue, stiff in-series and in-parallel elastic elements composed primarily of type I fibrillar collagen having the tensile strength of steel, each contributes to the progressive failure of this previously efficient muscular pump during systolic and/or diastolic phases of the cardiac cycle [40].

Previous myocardial infarction, hypertensive heart disease, or a dilated (idiopathic) cardiomyopathy may each contribute to the heart's failure as a muscular pump that is perpetuated by a sporadic and progressive necrosis of cardiomyocytes, replaced by fibrous tissue, and promoted by inappropriate neurohormonal activation and effector hormones of the rennin angiotensin aldosterone system and atrial natriuretic system. The hyperadrenergic, acute stressor state in congestive heart failure is accompanied by a translocation of K^+, Ca^{2+}, Mg^{2+}, and Zn^{2+} from the vascular to intracellular compartment. In the case of cardiac myocytes and mitochondria, intracellular Ca^{2+} overload and the induction of oxidative stress leads to mPTP opening, organellar degeneration, cardiomyocyte necrosis with myocardial fibrosis, and subsequent scarring. This Ca^{2+} paradox accounts for an induction of oxidative stress, leading to cardiomyocyte necrosis and subsequent reparative fibrosis. Fibrosis contributes to the adverse structural remodeling of the right and left heart with its attending pathologic influences on myocardial stiffness and contractility while it also serves as substrate for reentrant arrhythmias. An intrinsically coupled dyshomeostasis of Zn^{2+} and Se^{2+} is also seen, which compromises antioxidant defenses. Underlying the structural and geometric changes of remodeling, multiple cellular and molecular events must occur within the myocytes and the extracellular compartment. Most notably, a number of these events are induced and/or controlled by neurohormonal stimulation, which has been a major target of therapeutic pharmacological intervention. Chronic neurohormonal stimulation alters the contractile function of the cardiomyocyte by dysregulation of calcium metabolism within the cell [41]. Within the myocyte, the contractile structure is fundamentally changed by altering gene expression of contractile proteins, including myosin heavy chains by downregulation of alpha chains and upregulation of beta chains [42]. Myocyte death within the infarcted and non-infarcted myocardium plays an intricate role not only in the infarction expansion and thinning but also in the cell slippage in the non-infarcted myocardium, which allows longitudinal hypertrophy with resulting LV cavity dilation. Two methods of cell death have been documented: cell necrosis, and the more predominate mode of cell death, programmed cell death, called "apoptosis." Apoptosis occurs in the infarction and peri-infarction areas as well as in the remote myocardium; whereas necrosis occurs acutely in the infarction zone [43]. Apoptosis signaling appears to be coordinated by several factors: neurohormonal, cytokines, and extracellular triggers. After a myocyte dies, the remaining living cells are more able to "slip" because the number of viable cell–cell connections in the extracellular matrix is reduced.

Surrounding the myocytes, the extracellular matrix (ECM) is a dynamic complex composed of structural components: collagen, especially type I and III, and fibroblasts. More importantly, ECM is an active region, which coordinates cell–cell signaling molecules, namely, integrins, and contains within it zinc-dependent interstitial enzymatic proteins called "matrix metalloproteinases (MMPs)" and their tissue inhibitor counterparts, TIMPs. Integrins are mechanoreceptors on the myocyte cell membrane, which allow an intracellular biochemical response to extracellular mechanical stimuli, like stretch. MMPs are a collection of proenzymes that, when cleaved or activated, can perform a host of varied enzymatic activities. MMPs are critical players in the degradation of ECM, which allow cell movement and stimulate apoptotic pathways.[1]

The process of adverse ventricular remodeling needs to be understood both at the macroscopic and cellular level. The advent of pharmacological therapy targeting crucial steps in the molecular mechanisms holds promise if effectively translated

[1] With permission from Petra Kleinbongard. TNFα in myocardial ischemia/reperfusion, remodeling and heart failure. *Heart Failure Reviews* 2010;16(1). Copyright Springer science+ business media.

from the bench side to the bed side. However, in the scenario of advanced heart failure and advanced adverse remodeling, adjunctive therapy targeted at restoration of optimal ventricular form has a definitive role. To be able to address nontransplant surgery to each individual patient, a thorough understanding of ventricular remodeling following transmural myocardial infarctions is vital.

Therefore, the crux of adverse ventricular remodeling in ischemic or non-ischemic cardiomyopathy is the alterations in form which define the extent of altered function that profoundly impacts its various therapeutic modalities.

References

1. Buckberg GD, and The RESTORE group. Form versus disease: optimising geometry during ventricular restoration. Eur J Cardiothorac Surg. 2006;29: S238–44.
2. Tibayan FA, Lai DT, Timek TA, et al. Alterations in left ventricular torsion in tachycardia induced dilated cardiomyopathy. J Thorac Cardiovasc Surg. 2002;124: 43–9.
3. Spotniz MH. Macro design, structure and mechanics of the left ventricle. J Thorac Cardiovasc Surg. 2000;119(5):1053–77.
4. Coghlan C, Hoffman J. Leonardo da Vinci's flights of the mind must continue: cardiac architecture and the fundamental relation of form and function revisited. Eur J Cardiothorac Surg. 2006;29:S4–17.
5. Sallin EA. Fiber orientation and ejection fraction in the human ventricle. Biophys J. 1969;9:954–64.
6. Gould L, Lipscomb RK, Hamilton GW, Kennedy E. Relation of left ventricular shape, function and wall stress in man. Am J Cardiol. 1974;34:627–34.
7. Cohn JN, Ferrari R, Sharpe N. Cardiac remodeling—concepts and clinical implications: a consensus paper from an international forum on cardiac remodeling. J Am Coll Cardiol. 2000;35(3):569–82.
8. Whittaker P, Boughner DR, et al. Role of collagen in acute myocardial infarction expansion. Circulation. 1991;84:2123–34.
9. Hutchins GM, Bulkley BH. Infarct expansion versus extension. Two different complications of acute myocardial infarction. Am J Cardiol. 1978;41:1127–32.
10. Weisman HF, Bush DE, Mannisi JA, et al. Cellular mechanisms of myocardial infarction expansion. Circulation. 1988;78:186–201.
11. Pfeffer JM, Pfeffer MA, Fletcher PJ, Braunwald E. Progressive ventricular remodeling in rat with myocardial infarction. Am J Physiol. 1991;260 (5 Pt 2):H1406–14.
12. Olivetti G, Capasso JM, Sonnenblick EH, Anversa P. Side-to-side slippage of myocytes participates in ventricular wall remodeling acutely after myocardial infarction in rats. Circ Res. 1990;67(1):23–34.
13. McKay RG, Pfeffer MA, Pasternak RC, et al. Left ventricular remodeling following a myocardial infarction. A corollary to infarct expansion. Circulation. 1986;74:693–702.
14. Anand IS, Florea VG. Alterations in ventricular structure: role of left ventricular remodeling. In: Mann D, editor. Heart failure. Philadelphia: Saunders; 2004. p. 229–45.
15. Glower DD, Lowe JE. Left ventricular aneurysm. In: Cohn LH, Edmunds Jr LH, editors. Cardiac surgery in the adult. New York: McGraw-Hill; 2003. p. 771–88.
16. Kusakari Y, Xiaio CY, Himes N, Kinsella SD, Takahashi M, Rosenzweig A, Matsui T. Myocyte injury along myofibers in left ventricular remodeling after myocardial infarction. Interact Cardiovasc Thorac Surg. 2009;9:951–5.
17. Marino PN, Kass DA, Becker LC, et al. Influence of site of regional ischemia on nonischemic thickening in anesthetized dogs. Am J Physiol. 1989;25:H1417–25.
18. Erlebacher JA, Weiss JL, Weisfeldt ML, Bulkely BH. Early dilation of the infarcted segment in acute transmural myocardial infarction: role of infarct expansion in acute left ventricular enlargement. J Am Coll Cardiol. 1984;4:201–8.
19. Pirolo JS, Hutchins GM, Moore GW. Infarct expansion: pathologic analysis of 204 patients with a single myocardial infarct. J Am Coll Cardiol. 1986;7:349–54.
20. Radhakrishnan S, Ghista DN, Jayaraman G. Mechanics of left ventricular aneurysm. J Biomed Eng. 1986;8:9–23.
21. Rutherford JD, Braunwald E, Cohn PE. Chronic ischemic heart disease. In: Braunwald E, editor. Heart disease: a textbook of cardiovascular medicine. Philadelphia: WB Saunders; 1988. p. 1364.
22. Buckberg GD. Defining the relationship between akinesia and dyskinesia and the cause of left ventricular failure after anterior infarction and reversal of remodeling to restoration. J Thorac Cardiovasc Surg. 1998; 116:47–51.
23. de Oliveira JA. Heart aneurysm in Chagas' disease. Rev Inst Med Trop Sao Paulo. 1998;40:301–10.
24. Silverman KJ, Hutchins GM, Bulkley BH. Cardiac sarcoid: a clinicopathological study of 84 unselected patients with systemic sarcoidosis. Circulation. 1978;58:1204–9.
25. Davila JC, Enriquez F, Bergoglio S, et al. Congenital aneurysm of the left ventricle. Ann Thorac Surg. 1965;1:697–702.
26. Meizlish JL, Berger MJ, Plaukey M, et al. Functional left ventricular aneurysm formation after acute anterior transmural myocardial infarction: incidence, natural history, and prognostic implications. N Engl J Med. 1984;311:1001–11.
27. Forman MB, Collins HW, Kopelman HA, et al. Determinants of left ventricular aneurysm formation after anterior myocardial infarction: a clinical and angiographic study. J Am Coll Cardiol. 1986;8:1256–61.

28. Mills NL, Everson CT, Hockmuth DR. Technical advances in the treatment of left ventricular aneurysm. Ann Thorac Surg. 1993;55:792–811.
29. Glower DD, Schaper J, Kabas JS, et al. Relation between reversal of diastolic creep and recovery of systolic function after ischemic myocardial injury in conscious dogs. Circ Res. 1987;60:850–6.
30. Eaton LW, Weiss JL, Bulkley BH, et al. Regional cardiac dilation after acute myocardial infarction: recognition by two-dimensional echocardiography. N Engl J Med. 1979;300:57–63.
31. Markowitz LJ, Savage EB, Ratcliffe MB, et al. Large animal model of left ventricular aneurysm. Ann Thorac Surg. 1989;48:838–43.
32. Iwasaki K, Kita T, Taniguichi G, Kusachi S. Improvement of left ventricular aneurysm after myocardial infarction: report of three cases. Clin Cardiol. 1991;14:355–61.
33. Kayden DS, Wackers FJ, Zaret BL. Left ventricular aneurysm formation after thrombolytic therapy for anterior infarction. TIMI phase I and open label 1985–1986. Circulation. 1987;76 Suppl 4:97–101.
34. Chen JS, Hwang CL, Lee DY, et al. Regression of left ventricular aneurysm after delayed percutaneous transluminal coronary angioplasty (PTCA) in patients with acute myocardial infarction. Int J Cardiol. 1995;48:39–42.
35. Beltrami CA, Finato N, Rocco M, Feruglio GA, Puricelli C, Cigola E, Quaini F, Sonnenblick EH, Olivetti G, Anversa P. Structural basis of end-stage failure in ischemic cardiomyopathy in humans. Circulation. 1994;89:151–63.
36. Cotran RS, Kumar V, Robbins SL. The heart. In: Cotran RS, Kumar V, Robbins SL, editors. Robbins pathologic basis of disease. 4th ed. Philadelphia: WB Saunders; 1989. p. 597–656.
37. Park M, Shen YT, Gaussin V, Heyndrickx GR, Bartunek J, Resuello RR, Natividad FF, Kitsis RN, Vatner DE, Vatner SF. Apoptosis predominates in nonmyocytes in heart failure. Am J Physiol Heart Circ Physiol. 2009;297:H785–91.
38. Li H, Ambade A, Re F. Cutting edge: necrosis activates the NLRP3 inflammasome. J Immunol. 2009;183:1528–32.
39. Cohen I, Rider P, Carmi Y, Braiman A, Dotan S, White MR, Voronov E, Martin MU, Dinarello CA, Apte RN. Differential release of chromatin-bound IL-1α discriminates between necrotic and apoptotic cell death by the ability to induce sterile inflammation. Proc Natl Acad Sci USA. 2010;107:2574–9.
40. Weber KT. Cardiac interstitium in health and disease: the fibrillar collagen network. J Am Coll Cardiol. 1989;13:1637–52.
41. Lehnart SE, Maier LS, Hasenfuss G. Abnormalities of calcium metabolism and myocardial contractility depression in the failing heart. Heart Fail Rev. 2009;14(4):213–24.
42. Miyata S, Minobe W, Bristow MR, Leinwand LA. Myosin heavy chain iso-form expression in the failing and non-failing human heart. Circ Res. 2000;86:386–90.
43. Baldi A, Abbate A, Bussani R, Patti G, Melfi R, Angelini A, Dobrina A, Rossiello R, Silvestri F, Baldi F, Di Sciascio G. Apoptosis and post-infarction left ventricular remodeling. J Mol Cell Cardiol. 2002;34:165–74.

4 Altered Ventricular Function in Ischemic Cardiomyopathy

Introduction

The unique mode of left ventricular filling and ejection is by torsion in opposite directions, which is a function of its oblique myofibers. With occurrence of heart failure, irrespective of the underlying etiology, the torsion becomes suboptimal due to distortions in ventricular geometry. The alterations in ventricular geometry in ischemic cardiomyopathy have been detailed in the previous chapter. Here, we discuss about the various abnormalities of cardiac function in systole and diastole. Optimal function follows optimal form, as is evident by discussions in Chaps. 1 and 2. The perturbations in function which are the hallmark of ischemic cardiomyopathy with left ventricular aneurysms are detailed here.

As the normal LV inflow and outflow are in continuity, there is a need for torsion in systole to propel blood into the aorta, and a similar torsion in the opposite direction for negative suction during LV filling.

In the spherical dilated heart, due to horizontal orientation – "creep" of the fibers – both systole and diastole are affected. In diastole, the circumferential strain is reduced, leading to reduced amplitude of untwisting of the base. The negative suction vortex is not optimal with additional impairment in lengthening of the LV, leading to abnormal early filling.

During systole, the apical systolic torsion is reversed. The apex continues to rotate clockwise with reduction of maximum positive torsion. The maximum positive torsion is delayed until after end ejection. This signifies an increasing positive torsion during isovolumetric relaxation and early diastole, affecting both effective ventricular ejection and filling. As radial, circumferential, and longitudinal strains are also reduced, there is a nonuniformity of mean shear along the LV wall increasing wall stress. There is decreased longitudinal shortening of the lateral wall with systolic ascent instead of the normal descent of the mitral annulus [1]. In addition, there is abnormal stretching of the apex. The apex no longer retains its maximal curvature and hence is no longer an optimum fulcrum for ventricular contraction.

Myocardial Ischemia and Infarction

Left Ventricular Twist

In patients with anterior wall myocardial infarction, peak circumferential strain in the apex is significantly depressed in those patients with systolic dysfunction as compared with those with preserved systolic function [2]. The twist is severely depressed in presence of systolic dysfunction mainly due to reduced magnitude of apical rotation. With the onset of systolic dysfunction, the diastolic untwisting is also reduced and delayed [3]. In contrast, in those patients with anterior myocardial infarction and preserved left ventricular function, the systolic twist is preserved [3, 4]. In those patients with preserved systolic function, there is marginal reduction of apical circumferential strain and preservation of

V R. Parachuri, S.M. Adhyapak, *Ventricular Geometry in Post-Myocardial Infarction Aneurysms*,
DOI 10.1007/978-1-4471-2861-8_4, © Springer-Verlag London 2012

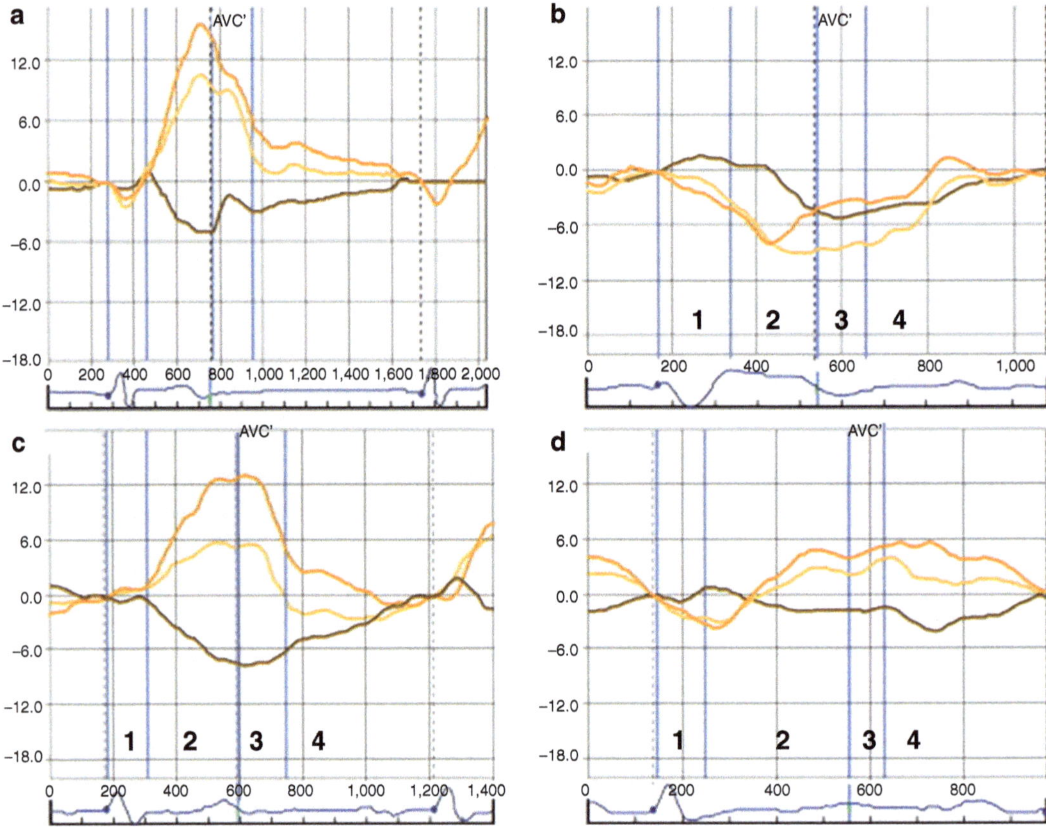

Fig. 4.1 LV twist in health and disease. Rotation of the left ventricular (LV) apex, the LV base, and the net LV twist angle (shown in *red*, *green*, and *black* colors, respectively) is assessed by speckle-tracking echocardiography in a normal subject (**a**), a patient with dilated cardiomyopathy with systolic heart failure (**b**), a patient with cardiac amyloidosis presenting as heart failure with normal ejection fraction (diastolic heart failure) (**c**), and a patient with constrictive pericarditis (**d**). Net ventricular twist is negative in dilated cardiomyopathy because of complete reversal of the LV apex rotation (**b**). In contrast, a patient with amyloid cardiomyopathy shows relatively preserved magnitude of net LV twist angle. In a normal subject, the onset of untwisting occurs just before the aortic valve closure (*AVC*) (**a**); however, in the patient with amyloid cardiomyopathy, the onset of untwisting is delayed after AVC (**c**). The patient with constrictive pericarditis (**d**) shows reduced magnitude of net ventricular twist and marked delay in the onset of untwisting (With permission from Sengupta et al. [7])

the apical twist. In patients with predominant subendocardial ischemia, there was greater than normal apical rotation, as rotation reflects subepicardial function which was preserved in these patients [5]. With transmural ischemia, there was less than normal apical rotation. In a study on normal subjects and patients with heart failure [6], it was noted that left ventricular ejection fraction correlated with apical but not with basal Rot_{max} (maximal rotation) (Fig. 4.1). Interestingly, in normal hearts, the LV sphericity index had a parabolic relation with apical Rot_{max} and $Twist_{max}$. A left ventricular sphericity index of ~2.1 was associated with the highest $Twist_{max}$; lower and higher sphericity indexes were associated with less $Twist_{max}$. Assuming that the LV sphericity index may be related to fiber orientation [8], a decreased LV sphericity index may be related to decreased $Twist_{max}$ due to a decreased fiber angle, whereas an increased LV sphericity index may be related to decreased $Twist_{max}$ as well, however, due to an increased fiber angle. In healthy volunteers, increased wall thickness, relative to the short-axis dimension of the LV cavity, was also associated with increased apical Rot_{max} and $Twist_{max}$. During the ejection phase, both the endocardial and epicardial spiraling fibers are electrically activated. However, the epicardial fibers govern the direction of LV twist, mainly owing to their longer arm of movement. It can therefore be anticipated that the epicardial fibers may become even more dominant when the LV walls are thicker, in particular relative to LV cavity dimension, because in such walls the differences in the arms of movement will be greater. The LV sphericity index, as a parameter of LV geometry, varied from 1.2 to 1.8 in DCM patients and showed a positive linear relation with apical Rot_{max} and $Twist_{max}$. Even when DCM patients with similar LV-EF were studied, the LV sphericity index remained positively correlated to both LV rotation parameters. In fact, the LV sphericity index was the strongest independent predictor of both apical Rot_{max} and $Twist_{max}$. Prevention of LV remodeling favorably impacts the untoward natural history of heart failure [9], which may be, at least partly, related to the preservation of LV twist. LV apical rotation and twist are significantly influenced by LV configuration. Taking the important function of LV twist into account, this finding highlights the vital influence of cardiac shape on LV systolic function.

Myocardial Strain

After transmural myocardial infarction, changes in intramural myocardial function will occur. Independent of localization, intramural deformation was found to be reduced in the infarcted myocardium. Therefore, the infarct area can be recognized by a specific spatial pattern of intramural deformation, including reduced and more circumferentially oriented systolic stretch (local systolic dilatation or bulging). Regional differences in intramural deformation between infarcted and noninfarcted (remote) myocardium were larger in the left anterior descending coronary artery related infarcts than circumflex or right coronary artery related infarcts of enzymatically the same size [10]. This finding may be one of the mechanical explanations of why anterior myocardial infarction seems more prone to postinfarct remodeling [11].

In a direct comparison between strain and wall thickening analysis, strain analysis was found to be superior in discriminating infarct from remote myocardium. For detecting dysfunctional myocardium, wall thickening analysis had a sensitivity of 69% and a specificity of 92%, whereas strain analysis showed a sensitivity of 92% and a specificity of 99%. The global ejection fraction correlated better with averaged myocardial strain ($r=0.89$, $p < 0.001$) than with wall thickening ($r=0.76$, $p < 0.005$) [12].

Some controversy exists about myocardial function in noninfarcted remote myocardium. In one study performed within 10 days after infarction, dysfunctional regions (infarcted myocardium), regions with normal function (adjacent myocardium), and regions with hypercontractile function (remote myocardium) were observed [13].

Another study, however, showed that patients with single-vessel disease had reduced intramyocardial circumferential shortening throughout the LV, including the remote noninfarcted regions on day 5 after first anterior infarction [14]. One explanation for these different findings might be the difference in definition of remote areas.

Eight weeks after first anterior infarction, strains remained reduced not only at the infarct area but also in the remote myocardium of the noninfarcted basal segment as well [15]. This persistent dysfunction in infarcted and noninfarcted areas may be one of the first indicators of progressive remodeling and the occurrence of heart failure late after myocardial infarction.

Ischemia also affects LV torsion and untwisting. In animal experiments, ischemia induced by a short period of coronary artery occlusion resulted in increased counterclockwise rotation. A probable explanation is the loss of counteraction of contraction of subendocardial, clockwise-oriented fibers because of subendocardial ischemia. When the occlusion persisted, the torsion pattern showed a form of pseudonormalization and finally was globally decreased, because contractility of subepicardial fibers also decreased [16]. A decrease in torsion was also observed in patients after myocardial infarction [17]. This reduction of torsion was related to the extent of the asynergic area and to a decrease of global ejection fraction.

Variations in Left Ventricular Twist with Onset of Ventricular Dilatation

As the ventricle dilates, the amplitude of peak left ventricular systolic twist is impaired in proportion to the global left ventricular function [18]. This reduction in left ventricular twist is accounted for by marked attenuation of left ventricular apical rotation with basal rotation being spared. In some patients, rotation of the apex may be abruptly interrupted such that in the initial part of systole, the left ventricular base and apex rotate in the same direction. After the initial part of systole, the rotation diverges into one of two patterns: either continuation of identical rotation at all levels for the remainder of systole or a divergence of rotation so that the apex and base rotate in opposite directions [19, 20].

Dilated Nonischemic Cardiomyopathy

In patients with nonischemic dilated cardiomyopathy (DCM), a consistent pattern of marked regional heterogeneity in myocardial function was found. In the septum, systolic lengthening (in both circumferential and longitudinal direction) instead of shortening was found during systole, whereas in the lateral wall, relatively normal systolic shortening occurred ($p < 0.001$ lateral vs. septal walls). Reduced function in the septal region may be related to increased wall stress, leading to relative hypoperfusion and subsequently myocardial dysfunction [21]. The normal left ventricular twist and left ventricular twist in various disease states have been delineated in Fig. 4.1.

In general, subendocardial hypoperfusion and concomitant reduced contraction in the subendocardium will lead to limited counteraction of clockwise rotation of the subepicardial fibers. This results in an increased net ventricular torsion. Importantly, decreased contractility and associated increased torsion as a result of hypoperfusion may occur far before irreversible tissue damage including increased collagen content and altered architecture becomes present [22–24] and thus may serve as early indicators of (reversible) cardiac abnormalities in patients prone to the development of structural cardiac damage and dysfunction.

Another factor contributing to heterogeneity in regional myocardial function in these patients might be the presence of conduction abnormalities. Dilated cardiomyopathy is often complicated by intraventricular conduction delay (25%), usually manifested as a left bundle branch block [25]. The presence of a left bundle branch block is associated with an asynchronous contraction pattern and worse outcome [26]. In a large population of patients with congestive heart failure, the presence of a left bundle branch block yielded a hazard ratio of 1.36 (95% confidence interval, 1.15–1.61, $p < 0.001$) for all-cause mortality.

Recently, CRT has emerged as a promising treatment strategy for this subgroup of heart failure patients [27]. However, approximately one-third of the patients eligible for CRT do not have response to this therapy [28], which raised the demand for adequate patient selection.

As shown by Nelson et al. [29] mechanical dyssynchrony is a key predictor for CRT efficacy in these patients. They quantified circumferential myocardial strain using MR tissue tagging in seven healthy subjects and eight patients with DCM and conduction delay before CRT, and measured the change in dP/dt_{max} during CRT. Circumferential shortening was significantly reduced in DCM hearts compared with control subjects ($-5.3 \pm 2.1\%$ vs. $-18.6 \pm 2.9\%$, $p < 0.001$), consistent with depressed myocardial function. In addition, a high variance in strain was observed in these patients ($201.4 \pm 84.3\%$ vs. $28.0 \pm 7.1\%$, $p < 0.001$), indicating a greater dispersion or heterogeneity of regional peak systolic strain. This indicator of mechanical dyssynchrony showed a good correlation with the change in dP/dt_{max} during CRT ($r = 0.85$, $p < 0.008$).

A study by Zwanenburg et al. [30] using MR tissue tagging with high temporal resolution (14 ms) showed that, in general, the onset of circumferential shortening in DCM patients propagated from the septum to the lateral wall, which is opposite to the direction found in normal subjects. However, in patients with nonischemic DCM, this pattern of mechanical activation was quite uniform, whereas in ischemic DCM, a wide range of directions of activation were found. As a consequence, the location of the area with delayed activation may vary as well, and this may be one of the mechanical explanations of why CRT is less effective in ischemic DCM [30].

Thus, nonischemic cardiomyopathy differs significantly from ischemic cardiomyopathy in terms of anatomical perturbations and functional perturbations. In ischemic cardiomyopathy, the alterations in apical geometry mainly define the altered torsion and ineffective systolic and diastolic function.

References

1. Helm PA, Younes L, Beg MF, Ennis DB, Leclerq C, Faris OP, Veigh EM, Kass D, Miller MI, Winslow RL. Evidence of structural remodeling in the dyssynchronous failing heart. Circ Res. 2006;98:125–32.
2. Gotte MJ, Van Rossum AC, Marcus JT, Kuijer JP, Axel L, Visser CA. Recognition of infarct localization by specific changes in intramural myocardial mechanics. Am Heart J. 1999;138:1038–41.
3. Takeyuchi M, Borden WB, Nakai IL. The assessment of left ventricular twist in anterior wall myocardial infarction using two dimensional speckle tracking imaging. J Am Soc Echocardiogr. 2007;20:36–44.
4. Garot J, Pascal O, Diebold B. Alterations of systolic left ventricular twist after acute myocardial infarction. Am J Physiol Heart Circ Physiol. 2002;282:H357–62.
5. Krocker CA, Tyberg JV, Beyar R. Effects of ischemia on left ventricular apex rotation: an experimental study in anaesthetized dogs. Circulation. 1995;92:3539–48.
6. van Dalen BM, Kauer F, Vletter WB, Soliman OII, van der Zwaan HB, ten Cate FJ, Geleijnse ML. Influence of cardiac shape on left ventricular twist. J Appl Physiol. 2010;108:1146–51.
7. Sengupta PP, Tajik AJ, Chandrasekaran K, Khandheria BK. Twist mechanics of the left ventricle: principles and application. JACC Cardiovasc Imaging. 2008;1:366–76.
8. Sengupta PP, Korinek J, Belohlavek M, Narula J, Vannan MA, Jahangir A, Khandheria BK. Left ventricular structure and function: basic science for cardiac imaging. J Am Coll Cardiol. 2006;48:1988–2001.
9. Mann DL, Acker MA, Jessup M, Sabbah HN, Starling RC, Kubo SH. Clinical evaluation of the CorCap Cardiac Support Device in patients with dilated cardiomyopathy. Ann Thorac Surg. 2007;84:1226–35.
10. Gotte MJ, van Rossum AC, Marcus JT, Kuijer JP, Axel L, Visser CA. Recognition of infarct localization by specific changes in intramural myocardial mechanics. Am Heart J. 1999;138:1038–41.
11. Holmes JW, Borg TK, Covell JW. Structure and mechanics of healing myocardial infarcts. Annu Rev Biomed Eng. 2005;7:223–53.
12. Gotte MJ, vanRossum AC, Twisk JWR, et al. Quantification of regional contractile function after infarction: strain analysis superior to wall thickening analysis in discriminating infarct from remote myocardium. J Am Coll Cardiol. 2001;37:808–81.
13. Marcus JT, Gotte MJ, vanRossum AC, et al. Myocardial function in infarcted and remote regions early after infarction in man: assessment by magnetic resonance tagging and strain analysis. Magn Reson Med. 1997;38:803–81.
14. Kramer CM, Rogers WJ, Theobald TM, Power TP, Petruolo S, Reichek N. Remote noninfarcted region dysfunction soon after first anterior myocardial infarction. A magnetic resonance tagging study. Circulation. 1996;94:660–6.
15. Kramer CM, McCreery CJ, Semonik L, et al. Global alterations in mechanical function in healed reperfused first anterior myocardial infarction. J Cardiovasc Magn Reson. 2000;2:33–41.
16. Kroeker CA, Tyberg JV, Beyar R. Effects of ischemia on left ventricular apex rotation. An experimental study in anesthetized dogs. Circulation. 1995;92:3539–48.
17. Garot J, Pascal O, Diebold B, et al. Alterations of systolic left ventricular twist after acute myocardial infarction. Am J Physiol Heart Circ Physiol. 2002;282: H357–62.
18. Kanzaki H, Nakatani S, Yamada N. Impaired systolic torsion in dilated cardiomyopathy: reversal of apical rotation at mid systole characterized with magnetic resonance tagging method. Basic Res Cardiol. 2006;101:465–70.
19. Setser RM, Kasper JM, Lieber ML. Persistent abnormal left ventricular systolic torsion in dilated cardiomyopathy after partial left ventriculotomy. J Thorac Cardiovasc Surg. 2003;126:48–55.
20. Setser RM, Smedira NG, Lieber ML, Sabo ED, White RD. Left ventricular torsion mechanics after left ventricular reconstruction surgery for ischemic cardiomyopathy. J Thorac Cardiovasc Surg. 2007;134:888–96.
21. van den Heuvel AF, van Veldhuisen DJ, van der Wall EE, et al. Regional myocardial blood flow reserve impairment and metabolic changes suggesting myocardial ischemia in patients with idiopathic dilated cardiomyopathy. J Am Coll Cardiol. 2000;35:19–28.
22. Villari B, Cambell SE, Hess OM, et al. Influence of collagen network on left ventricular systolic and diastolic function in aortic valve disease. J Am Coll Cardiol. 1993;22:1477–84.
23. Gallagher KP, Osakada G, Hess O, Koziol JA, Kemper WS, Ross J. Subepicardial segmental function during coronary stenosis and the role of myocardial fiber orientation. Circ Res. 1982;50:352–9.
24. Prinzen FW, Arts T, Hoeks APG, Reneman RS. Discrepancies between myocardial blood flow and fiber shortening in the ischemic border zone as assessed with video mapping of epicardial deformation. Pflugers Arch. 1989;415:220–9.
25. Murkofsky RL, Dangas G, Diamond JA, Mehta D, Schaffer A, Ambrose JA. A prolonged QRS duration on surface electrocardiogram is a specific indicator of

left ventricular dysfunction. J Am Coll Cardiol. 1998;32:476–82.
26. Baldasseroni S, Opasich C, Gorini M, et al. Left bundle-branch block is associated with increased 1-year sudden and total mortality rate in 5517 outpatients with congestive heart failure: a report from the Italian network on congestive heart failure. Am Heart J. 2002;143:398–405.
27. Kass DA. Ventricular resynchronization: pathophysiology and identification of responders. Rev Cardiovasc Med. 2003;4 Suppl 2:S3–13.
28. Reuter S, Garrigue S, Barold SS, et al. Comparison of characteristics in responders versus nonresponders with biventricular pacing for drug-resistant congestive heart failure. Am J Cardiol. 2002;89:346–50.
29. Nelson GS, Curry CW, Wyman BT, et al. Predictors of systolic augmentation from left ventricular preexcitation in patients with dilated cardiomyopathy and intraventriculair conduction delay. Circulation. 2000;101:2703–9.
30. Zwanenburg JJM, Gotte MJW, Marcus JT, et al. Propagation of onset and peaktime of myocardial shortening in time of myocardial shortening in ischemic versus nonischemic cardiomyopathy: assessment by magnetic resonance imaging myocardial tagging. J Am Coll Cardiol. 2005;46:2215–22.

5 Hemodynamics in Ischemic Cardiomyopathy: Left Ventricular Aneurysm Formation

Introduction

The sequence of aneurysm formation and its effects on altered cardiac function in ischemic cardiomyopathy have been detailed in the previous chapters. It is vital to understand the hemodynamics of cardiac function and its consequences on cardiac homeostasis to plan therapeutic strategies to combat the adverse effects of ischemic cardiomyopathy. This chapter discusses the hemodynamic consequences of ineffective torsion due to horizontal orientation of oblique myofibers in the dilated heart. Cardiac dilatation follows large areas of myocardial scar which are sequelae of transmural myocardial infarctions. The alterations in systolic and diastolic function as a result of increased wall stress impact profoundly on mortality and morbidity. The area of scar tissue is a critical determinant of cardiac function.

The fibrotic scar formation in the left ventricular wall following a transmural myocardial infarction is usually located along the midmyocardium, rather than the endomyocardium or epimyocardium [1]. Magnetic resonance studies have demonstrated a significant decrease in percent wall thickening in the border and remote zones of the infarct area. The scar extension also tends to be confined to the midmyocardium. This scar extension is a critical predictor of adverse ventricular remodeling in the chronic phase. This midmyocardial location of scar strongly supports the presence of the helical myofiber band.

Factors Determining the Bulging of a Ventricular Aneurysm

After a transmural infarction, a well-delineated area of nonuniform interstitial fibrosis develops which can increasingly bulge outward during systole [2]. This constitutes a ventricular aneurysm. Its formation depends on the strength of the scar tissue and on traction forces acting on this tissue [3]. As the structural changes after myocardial infarction slowly increase myocardial stiffness during scar formation, the aneurysm gradually expands over a period of 4–6 weeks [4]. The clinical outcome of left ventricular aneurysms with or without repair is related to the size of the aneurysm, which is quantified by the left ventricular end-diastolic volume. However, size alone may not be a predictor of further enlargement. From a purely mechanistic view, neglecting myocardial ischemia, tissue characteristics, and elastic properties of both the aneurismal and nonaneurismal portions, both bradycardia and tachycardia are detrimental for aneurysm expansion. A heart rate of approximately 80 beats/minute might minimize bulging and the underlying forces acting on the aneurismal ventricular wall. The factors influencing wall stress in an aneurysm are varied. End-systolic wall stress of the aneurysm is markedly influenced by ventricular contractility and to a lesser extent by ventricular ejection. The relationship between afterload and aneurismal wall stress is not as strong as between after load and volume of the bulging area. This is

V R. Parachuri, S.M. Adhyapak, *Ventricular Geometry in Post-Myocardial Infarction Aneurysms*,
DOI 10.1007/978-1-4471-2861-8_5,

consistent with the observation that there is a weak relation between contractility and extent of bulging and limited correlation between contractility and aneurysm wall velocity during the cardiac cycle. Preload is only of secondary importance to aneurysm bulging. The afterload is more closely related to bulging and ventricular output due to formation of an aneurysm. This logarithmic relation clearly shows that afterload reduction would dramatically reduce bulging. In contrast, bulging is difficult to avoid with increasing systemic vascular resistance. This fact is consistent with clinical results of angiotensin-converting-enzyme inhibitors, decreasing the 4–6-week mortality and improving left ventricular function following myocardial infarctions [5–7].

Klein et al. [8] studied patients with left ventricular aneurysms by ventriculography. The aneurysms seen in the prethombolytic era and prior to percutaneous transluminal coronary angioplasty comprised of mainly fibrous tissue which was increasingly compliant, resulting in paradoxical expansion in systole or dyskinetic aneurysms. However, with reperfusion establishing patency of the infarct-related artery, the aneurismal wall may not be completely fibrotic, but may contain islands of viable myocardium with relatively preserved myocardial thickness. If the myocardium at the border zone of the aneurysm is injured or rather ischemic, the onset or height of tension development is delayed, and this portion of myocardium would stretch under the influence of greater tension developed in the remote myocardium.

This results in two consequences:

First, during active contraction, blood may be selectively transferred into the aneurismal sac, simulating mitral insufficiency and vitiating aortic ejection.

Second, the rate of development of tension in the composite left ventricle is slowed because the slack aneurysm acts as an elastic element in series with the contractile element. The slackness in the elastic component requires either faster or more extensive shortening of the contractile component to generate tension in isovolumic systole. Hence, much of the myocardial shortening is expended in generating tension with little reserve left for expulsion of blood. This elastic effect accounts for the markedly slow rate of rise of pressure during isovolumic systole.

If an aneurysm is predominantly akinetic and rigid, it may "splint" the normal cardiac wall during contraction and dissipate the inward vector of circumferential shortening. Although these aneurysms did not bulge during systole, there may be an imperceptible elastic stretch at the border zones. Thus there may be a continuum between pure dyskinesia and pure akinesia as mechanical defects in the dynamics of an aneurysm during the cardiac cycle.

Surface Area of the Aneurysm

When aneurysmal area approached 20–25% of the surface area of the left ventricle, the extent of shortening required of the remaining functioning heart has to exceed physiological limits (approximately 30% of maximum initial muscle length). As a consequence, stroke volume must fall.

This situation may be further aggravated by two considerations.

1. The involved area may not only be nonfunctioning but may also expand paradoxically.

   Because of the translocation of blood during systole, this will further increase the mechanical burden resulting from any given amount of immobile surface.
2. The functioning muscle itself is often afflicted, to varying degrees, with the underlying ischemic process and may be unable to compensate effectively.

Other possible mechanisms adversely affecting stroke volume:

1. Mitral incompetence.
2. Atrioventricular asynergy: Normal papillary muscle function is considered important not only to close the mitral valve but also to prime isovolumic contraction. Several aneurysms are so situated, so as to interfere with anterior papillary muscle function.
3. Asynchrony: The temporal sequence of contraction influences ventricular performance profoundly.

Quantification of Myocardial Involvement in Relation to Cardiac Dilatation

Left ventricular end-diastolic volume was markedly increased when the aneurysm comprised 20–25% of the ventricular surface area. This fact had broad implications. For the first time, it has been possible to quantify the degree of heart disease leading to ventricular dilatation. Just as a critical mitral or aortic valve size exists beyond which transvalvular flow cannot be increased owing to physiological limitations in pressure-generating capacity, so also a critical aneurysm size exists beyond which stroke output cannot be maintained because of physiological limitations in myocardial fiber shortening capacity.

When 20–25% of ventricular surface area becomes akinetic, dilatation must ensue if the limits of fiber shortening of healthy myocardium are not to be exceeded.

Inadequate Hemodynamic Compensation

According to the Frank–Starling hypothesis, increased ventricular size should lead to increased stroke volume and effective work within physiological constraints. Composite shortening in an aneurismal ventricle equalled only 5% of initial length, and hence, stroke volume was reduced, although the left ventricle was large. Since large areas of ventricular surface area remain virtually immobile throughout systole, regional changes in circumferential fiber shortening of healthy muscle ranged from 6% to 12% in the study of left ventricular aneurysms by Klein [8]. This being far less than the 12–18% observed in normal subjects at rest.

Despite ventricular dilatation acting geometrically to expel more blood for the same degree of shortening and also to augment contraction, myocardial decompensation was clearly evident. The very increase in heart size occasioned by dilatation and deformation of the aneurysm increases the radius of curvature of the ventricle and, hence, myocardial systolic tension requirements (average two to two-and-a-half times normal), but only a portion of the myocardium is available to respond to increased stretch. The effects of afterload to inhibit ejection may have exceeded the effects of preload to increase it forcing dilatation of the un infarcted portions of the left ventricle.

Theoretical Force-Velocity-Length Considerations

A contractile element (CE) in series with an undamped series elastic element (SEE), which has a force-dependent stiffness, is used to theoretically explain the force velocity muscle fiber length considerations during the cardiac cycle [9]. Muscle contraction involves stretching of the SEE by the CE during force generation (isometric contraction) and subsequent shortening of the fiber during continued CE shortening (auxotonic contraction). A fundamental characteristic governing contraction is the inverse force-velocity relationship at any given length. A dilated left ventricle requires increased wall tension to maintain a given pressure. Less contractile element shortening, however, is required because the force-dependent SEE is stretched faster and more blood is ejected per unit shortening at a larger size.

Not only is the absolute force increased in the patient with aneurysm and cardiac dilatation, but the time course of the systolic load is shifted. Unlike the normal left ventricle where force begins to decline about 80 ms after inception of systolic ejection, the ventricle with aneurysm labors with a progressively increasing force throughout two-thirds of systole. This is further aggravated if, in addition, the aneurysm acts as a compliant series elastic element. At the same time, instantaneous volume and, therefore, fiber length are decreasing (however little), as blood is ejected from the heart. Consequently, the ventricle shifts to progressively less effective force-velocity curves, and contractile element velocity is further inhibited.

Therefore, the prolonged time course of the systolic load associated with ventricular aneurysm will tend to reduce CE shortening and power, quite apart from the absolute elevation in mean systolic force. The course of force development depends on the speed of onset of active state as well as the CE-SEE interrelationships. For heart muscle, the onset and decline of the active state are time-dependent with maximum intensity attained at, or shortly before, the point of maximum isometric force and with a slow subsequent decline. The active state has been assessed in terms of velocity of shortening, correlated with time elapsed between resting and peak isometric tension, and equated with maximum d*p*/d*t*, the rate of isometric pressure change.

Striking reductions in d*p*/d*t* are seen particularly in patients with large aneurysms, signifying a reduced average rate of tension development of the composite left ventricle. This could arise from any of the following factors: (1) the series' elastic effect of slackness of the aneurysm, (2) variation in regional instantaneous wall tension resulting in contraction in one area and expansion in another, and (3) reduction in the maximally achieved intensity of the active state.

Mechanics of Left Ventricular Aneurysm Formation

An acute infarct has very low stiffness, and if it involves the entire wall, there is a risk of rupture: however, in the absence of such a critical situation, fibrous tissue is laid into the infarcted myocardial segment. Such an infarcted fibrotic myocardial segment will not be able to contract and so generate tensile stress. The surrounding intact myocardium will contract and generate wall stress, thereby developing a high intrachamber systolic pressure; the chronically infarcted and fibrotic segment will have to sustain this high chamber pressure. Its loss of contractility and the resulting reduced systolic stiffness relative to the intact segment will cause it to deform into a bulge, which is an aneurysm.

To determine the left ventricular wall deformation and the stress arising from infarction of a wall segment (which leads to a ventricular aneurysm), the left ventricle was modeled as a pressurized ellipsoidal shell. Deformations of infarcted wall segments were computed for several damaged wall thicknesses in left ventricles of different shapes. The analysis involved a derivation of equations for wall-stress equilibrium with the chamber pressure and myocardial incompressibility before and after infarct formation.

The dependence of tensile stress and the bulge of infarcted wall segments, on the extent of damaged wall thickness and the angle of infarct, were computed.

The percentage of infarcted wall thickness and the shape of the ellipsoidal left ventricular chamber played more dominant roles than the angle of damage or the extent of the infarct [10].

Ventricular Efficiency in the Failing Heart

The concept of mechanical efficiency of the heart as an index of overall cardiac performance was first introduced by Evans and Matsuka [11]. They observed that in Starling heart-lung preparations, the efficiency values decreased as progressive cardiac dilatation ensued. They also made the important discovery that cardiac efficiency was greater during high volume loads than during high pressure loads.

The term mechanical efficiency implies that it is a fundamental variable of pump performance which is representative of the fraction of total energy consumed which is converted into useful work. It can be determined by measuring the external work performed by the ventricle and its energy expenditure. Left ventricular minute work is calculated from the product of stroke volume, heart rate, and mean systolic left ventricular pressure. Myocardial energy expenditure can be equated with myocardial oxygen consumption, because the metabolism of the heart is almost exclusively aerobic in the absence of acute ischemia.

In heart failure, left ventricular efficiency is severely decreased, reflecting reduced work performance and high myocardial oxygen consumption. There is reduction of ejection phase indices and left ventricular stroke volume. Due to decreases in left ventricular systolic pressure and stroke volume, the left ventricular stroke work and work per minute are also decreased. Although the left ventricular mass is increased, the mean left ventricular myocardial blood flow is decreased. The mechanical efficiency is therefore reduced in this clinical scenario. The ejection phase indices of left ventricular function including ejection fraction, mean velocity of circumferential fiber shortening, stroke power index, and percent chordal shortening all correlate positively with left ventricular mechanical efficiency. This reflects on the fact that ventricular efficiency is calculated from ventricular work performance which is largely determined by the contractile state of the ventricle [12].

Effect of Ventricular Dilatation on the Stroke Volume (SV) in the Failing Ventricle Extension of the Frank–Starling Mechanism in the Failing Heart

The geometrical determinants of cardiac SV have been evaluated on the basis of mathematical models of the left ventricle [13].

It has been found that despite increasing wall stress, the SV generally increases with increasing anatomical cardiac size, reaching a maximum beyond which it decreases. On the basis of a model of a thick-walled sphere representing the left ventricle, SV relations have been computed for three different types of chronic ventricular enlargement. The three models are that of concentric hypertrophy, eccentric hypertrophy, and predominant increases of ventricular volume without hypertrophy. In all three models, the SV increases correlated only with increasing ventricular size up to a certain size and decreased as the size was increased further. Thus, it was hypothesized that the SV can be augmented with increasing ventricular size, under constant contractility despite decreasing ejection fractions [13]. Here, the slope of the curve describing the relation between SV and anatomical ventricular size was flattened, and the maximum of the curve was shifted toward smaller end-diastolic volumes in the presence of reduced contractility, distensibility, or after loss of contractile tissue. Human studies of heart failure have shown that pumping failure occurs when the ventricular operating point has reached the maximum, so that compensation by increase in ventricular size has been exhausted [14–17]. This hypothesis is an extension of the Frank–Starling mechanism operating in ischemic cardiomyopathy, where the SV increases with increasing end-diastolic volume (EDV) beyond the normal EDV limit, with decreasing contractility and decreasing ejection fraction. This mechanism is explained by the increased sensitivity of the calcium channels in the existing contractile myocardium [16, 17]. When a certain magnitude of EDV is reached, that is the point of maximal compensation of the SV to increases in EDV, the SV begins to decline. This decline in SV is related to the degree of left ventricular dilatation only and not related to the presence of compensatory remodeling. At this point, the sensitivity of calcium channels in the contractile myocardium also begins to decline.

This hypothesis has been validated clinically in our patients. In our patients, only the indexed end-diastolic volume (EDVI) and ejection fraction (EF) were related in significant linear relationships with the indexed stroke volume (SVI) (Fig. 5.1). The indexed stroke volume (SVI) had a significant linear relationship with the LV EF (Fig. 5.2). The SVI in our patients increased proportional to increases in EDVI in patients with EDVI ≤ 150 mL in conjunction with reduced EF. In patients with EDVI ≥ 150 mL, the SVI decreased and had no relationship with the EDVI. The patients with EDVI > 150 mL had significantly larger left ventricles as compared to the patients with EDVI < 150 mL. Thus, in our patients, the maximal ventricular operating point was an EDVI > 150 mL. Their EF was greater, and the SVI was lesser than patients with smaller left ventricles, but the difference was not statistically significant. The magnitude of EDVI at the maximal ventricular operating point in relation to increments in SVI for each individual patient, beyond which the SVI declines, may vary.

In the normal heart under various physiological loading conditions, the indexed end-systolic volume (ESVI) bears a significant linear relationship to the EF [18]. In our patients, there was no significant relationship between ESVI and SVI,

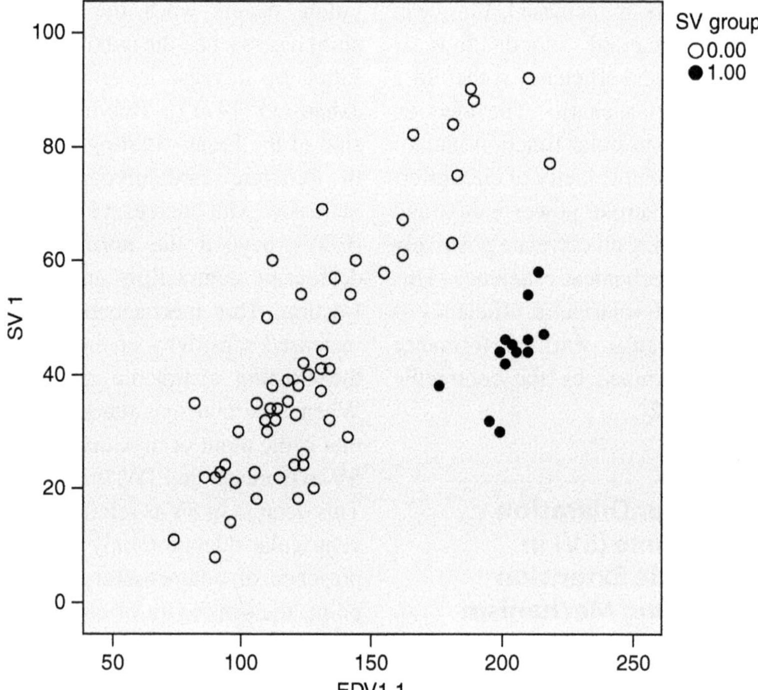

Fig. 5.1 Relationship of EDVI and SVI at baseline. Marker 0 (*clear circles*) –Patients who demonstrated increase in SV with increasesin EDV at baseline, Marker 1 (*black circles*) – Patients who did not demonstrate an increase in SV at baseline with increases in EDV (With permission from Adhyapak SM, Parachuri VR. Impact of surgical ventricular restoration on the stroke volume: surgical fine tuning of the relationship between end diastolic volume and stroke volume. J Thorac Cardiovasc Surg. 2011;141(6):1552–3. Copyright Elsevier)

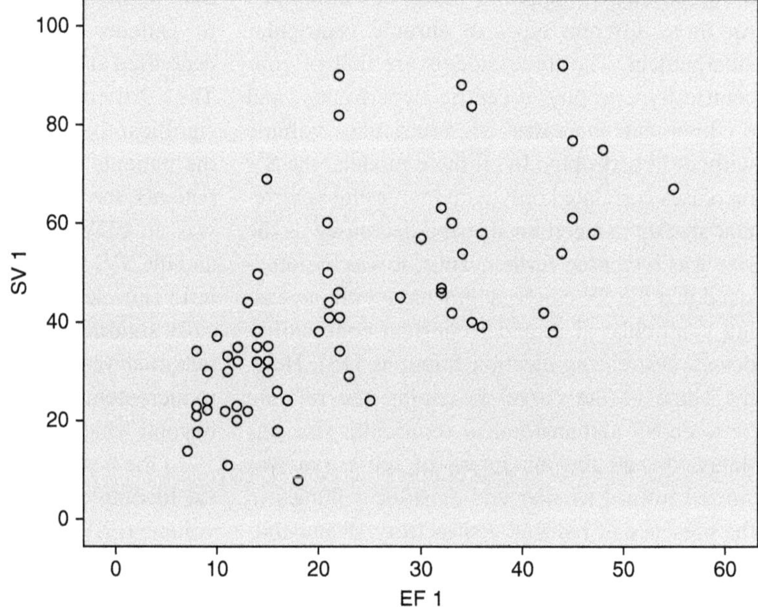

Fig. 5.2 Relationship of EF and SVI at baseline

and ESVI and EF. The reason for this phenomenon could be that in the course of remodeling, the dilated LV attempts to compensate by decreasing its ESVI to maintain an effective cardiac output, and hence, the ESVI may not be significantly related to its stroke volume or EF.

Effect of Geometric Remodeling Patterns on the SV Effect of Preload and Afterload

While studying the effect of preload and afterload on the SV, we studied the two geometric remodeling patterns of eccentric hypertrophy and concentric remodeling. The pattern of eccentric hypertrophy was the substrate for preload, and the pattern of concentric remodeling was the substrate for afterload. The pattern of eccentric hypertrophy most likely reflects the increase in venous return that, in the absence of an increase in peripheral needs, depends on an increase in circulatory mass, which in turn depends on water and sodium retention. In other words, eccentric remodeling identifies a "backward heart failure" secondary to the increase in filling pressure with pulmonary congestion. This factor is rarely taken into account when pressure-volume loops of ventricles with different geometries are compared. In our study, the patients with eccentric hypertrophy had significantly greater LV EDVI and ESVI with lesser EF, signifying greater degrees of LV dilatation than patients with concentric remodeling. The EF was better preserved in the concentric remodeling group. The presence of both concentric remodeling and eccentric hypertrophy had no significant effect on the SVI.

The mathematical model studies of Gulch and coworkers [13], where perturbations in the preload or afterload seen as representative forms of ventricular remodeling patterns of eccentric hypertrophy and concentric remodeling, have no effect on the SVI in heart failure and beyond the maximal ventricular operating point, only increases in EDVI cause decreases in SV [13–15], stand clinically validated.

In left ventricular aneurysms, inhomogeneity of ventricular contraction and relaxation is reflected as mechanical intraventricular dyssynchrony.

Intraventricular Mechanical Dyssynchrony

The myocardial scar leads to tissue inhomogeneity of dyskinetic and akinetic muscle, where nonuniform contraction, relaxation, and filling may develop and contribute to deterioration of global systolic and diastolic function. This intraventricular dyssynchrony stems from asynchrony of the component parts of the left ventricular chamber and may be independent of electrical conduction delay.

Here, mechanical events such as early and late shortening, early and late relaxation, or lengthening reflect interacting areas of differing performance of myocardium, which are considered irreversible. Conversely, during ischemia, similar abnormalities are linked to afterload increase and become reversible when blood supply is restored [19, 20].

Systolic lengthening occurs during the isovolumic phase and is caused by stretching of ischemic/scarred adjacent segments by the normally contracting segments seen in aneurysms. Energy is expended as normal segments contract to produce pressure, because tensile strength is required. The ischemic/scarred segment is unable to generate sufficient tension and thus passively bulges. The consequence is dissipation and wasting of some energy produced by normal segments, which stretch the ischemic/scarred tissue and therefore does not contribute to ejection [21]. These changes explain the impaired mechanical synchrony, which define global function.

Patients with ischemic cardiomyopathy were studied using pressure-volume loops for intraventricular mechanical dyssynchrony by Marisa Di Donato et al. [22]. Most pressure-volume loops showed abnormalities in morphology, size, and orientation. The most common observed abnormalities were early shortening and early relaxation, with markedly reduced effective work. Early shortening occurs because of the unloading effect of dyskinetic myocardium in series, which acts as an elastic slack element during the isovolumic phase of contraction [23]. Right-oriented loops were observed at the anteroapical regions. This type of loop abnormality meant the loss of all contractile properties. Paradoxical systolic expansion meant absence of force development and stretching by adjacent normal fibers. Early shortening and early lengthening were experimentally reproducible by connecting weak and strong myocardium in series [24]. Thus, within one cardiac cycle, regional pressure-volume loops moved in an opposite direction and asynchronously, giving each region a different contribution to global ejection.

These mechanical dyssynchrony indices were independent of electrical dyssynchrony which is evident by the presence of intraventricular conduction delay on the surface electrocardiogram. In those patients who demonstrate a left bundle branch block, biventricular pacing or cardiac resynchronization therapy has its benefits. These patients with left bundle branch block demonstrated both electrical and mechanical dyssynchrony. The pathogenesis of electromechanical dyssynchrony is beyond the confines of this chapter.

Thus, several factors play a role in adverse ventricular remodeling. The surface area of the ventricular scar being critical in determining the degree of ventricular dilatation leading to adverse hemodynamics which ultimately causes a steep decline, despite various compensatory mechanisms acting in concert to resurrect the failing cardiac pump.

References

1. Kusakari Y, Xiaio CY, Hines N, Kinsella SD, Takahashi M, Rosenweig A, Matsui T. Myocyte injury along myofibers in left ventricular remodelling after myocardial infarction. Interact Cardiovasc Thorac Surg. 2009;9:951–5.
2. Matsumoto M, Watanabe F, Goto A, et al. Left ventricular aneurysm and the prediction of left ventricular enlargement studied by two-dimensional echocardiography: quantitative assessment of aneurysm size in relation to clinical course. Circulation. 1985;72:280–6.
3. Moulton MJ, Downing SW, Creswell LL, et al. Mechanical dysfunction in the border zone of an ovine model of left ventricular aneurysm. Ann Thorac Surg. 1995;60:986–97.
4. Kleiger RE, Miller JP, Thanavaro S, Province MA, Martin TF, Oliver GC. Relationship between clinical features of acute myocardial infarction and ventricular runs 2 weeks to 1 year after infarction. Circulation. 1981;63:64–70.
5. The Acute Infarction Ramipril Efficacy (AIRE) Study Investigators. Effect of ramipril on mortality and morbidity of survivors of acute myocardial infarction with clinical evidence of heart failure. Lancet. 1993;342:821–8.
6. Gruppo Italiano per lo Studio della Sopravvivenza nell'infarto Miocardico. The GISSI-3: effects of lisinopril and transdermal glyceryl trinitrate singly and together on 6-week mortality and ventricular function after acute myocardial infarction. Lancet. 1994;343:1115–22.
7. Bartel T, Vanheiden H, Schaar J, Mertzkirch W, Erbel R. Biomechanical modelling of hemodynamic factors determining bulging of ventricular aneurysms. Ann Thorac Surg. 2002;74:1581–7.
8. Klein MD, Herman MV, Gorlin R, Vayo HW. A hemodynamic study of left ventricular aneurysm. Circulation. 1967;35:614–30.
9. Sonnenblick EH. Determinants of the active state in heart muscle: force-velocity, instantaneous muscle length, time. Fed Proc. 1965;24:1396–407.
10. Radhakrishnan S, Ghista DN, Jayaraman G. Mechanics of left ventricular aneurysm. J Biomed Eng. 1986;8:9–23.
11. Evans CL, Matsuoka Y. The effect of various mechanical conditions on the gaseous metabolism and efficiency of the mammalian heart. J Physiol. 1915;49:378–405.
12. Nichols AB, Pearson MH, Sciacca RR, Cannon PJ. Left ventricular mechanical efficiency in coronary artery disease. J Am Coll Cardiol. 1986;7:270–9.
13. Gulch RW, Jacob R. Geometric and muscle physiologic determinants of cardiac stroke volume as evaluated on the basis of model calculations. Basic Res Cardiol. 1988;83:476–85.
14. Jacob R, Dierberger B, Gulch RW, Kissling G. Geometric and muscle physiologic factors of the Frank–Starling mechanism. Basic Res Cardiol. 1993;88:86–91.
15. Jacob R, Gulch RW. The functional significance of ventricular geometry for the transition from hypertrophy to cardiac failure. Does a critical degree of structural dilatation exist? Basic Res Cardiol. 1998;93:423–9.
16. Holubarsch C, Ruf T, Goldstein DJ, Ashto RC, Nickl W, Pieske B, Pioch K, Ludemann J, Weissner S, Hasenfuss G, Poseval H, Just H, Burkhoff D. Existence of the Frank–Starling mechanism in the failing human heart. Circulation. 1996;94:683–9.
17. Mangano DT, Van Dyke DC, Ellis RJ. The effect of increasing preload on ventricular output and ejection in man. Limitations of the Frank–Starling mechanism. Circulation. 1980;62:535–41.
18. Renlund DG, Gerstenblith G, Fleg JL, Becker LC, Lakatta EG. Interaction between end diastolic and end systolic volumes in normal humans. Am J Physiol Heart Circ Physiol. 1990;258:H473–81.
19. Tyberg JV, Forrester JS, Wyatt HL, et al. An analysis of segmental ischemic dysfunction utilizing pressure-length loop. Circulation. 1974;49:748–54.

20. Theroux AW, Franklin D, Ross Jr J, et al. Regional myocardial function during acute coronary occlusion and its modification by pharmacologic agents in the dog. Circ Res. 1974;35:896–908.
21. Safwat A, Leone BJ, Norris RM, et al. Pressure-length loop area: its components analyzed during graded myocardial ischemia. J Am Coll Cardiol. 1991;17:790–6.
22. Di Donato M, Toso A, Dor V, Sabatier M, Barletta G, Menicanti L, Fantini F, and the RESTORE group. Surgical ventricular restoration improves mechanical intraventricular dyssynchrony in ischemic cardiomyopathy. Circulation. 2004;109:2536–43.
23. Sasayama S, Nonogi H, Fujita M, et al. Analysis of asynchronous wall motion by regional pressure-length loops in patients with coronary artery disease. J Am Coll Cardiol. 1984;4:259–67.
24. Wiegner AW, Allen GJ, Bing OHL. Weak and strong myocardium in series: implications for segmental dysfunction. Am J Physiol. 1978;235:H776–83.

Evolution of Techniques of Surgical Ventricular Restoration: From Linear Repair to Endoventricular Linear Patch Plasty

6

Introduction

The first two chapters have focused on the normal ellipsoid ventricular architecture, its myofiber organization, and its unique mode of filling and ejection. With the advent of diseases like transmural myocardial infarction, scar formation, and subsequent ventricular dilatation, the perturbations in anatomy and function have also been detailed. It is essential for cardiac surgeons to comprehend the central theme of that of altering structure effects function profoundly. This concept forms the basis of surgical restoration of dilated, distorted ventricles of patients in advanced congestive cardiac failure. The knowledge of ventricular structures helps impact surgical decisions concerning operative modifications in restoring a near physiological form, which are delicately balanced on the interplay of left ventricular spatial relationships. Early reperfusion procedures for acute myocardial infarction, whether by thrombolysis or angioplasty, have altered the pathological changes that follow acute myocardial infarction.

Reperfusion produces epicardial and, occasionally, mid-myocardial sparing while leaving endocardial necrosis. Persistence of viable ventricular muscle frequently trades left ventricular dyssynergy for asynergy, with some preservation of wall thickness. When one third or more of the ventricular perimeter is involved, left ventricular volume markedly increases, the apical and basal portions become rounded, and pump function is globally depressed. This condition resembles dilated nonischemic cardiomyopathy more than classic dyskinetic aneurysm.

Ventricular Dilatation

The underlying ischemic insult ranges from an extensive post-myocardial infarction scar leading to secondary stretch of compensatory remote fibers within unscarred myocardium or global stretch from multiple small scars, but without a large region of asynergy.

The ventricular enlargement into a dilated sphere forms a unifying theme for the downward spiral of associated pathological abnormalities which conspire to cause adverse remodeling and a potentially inexorable decline toward intractable congestive cardiac failure. Therefore, ventricular volume should be reduced in its septal and anterior components without deforming the ventricular chamber.

Secondary Changes in the Mitral Apparatus

The ventricular stretch alters mitral leaflet coaptation. The mitral annulus also widens secondary to dilatation of the cardiac base. The resulting widening of the distance between papillary muscle bases amplifies leaflet tethering and further limits their coaptation.

V R. Parachuri, S.M. Adhyapak, *Ventricular Geometry in Post-Myocardial Infarction Aneurysms*,
DOI 10.1007/978-1-4471-2861-8_6,

Revascularization

Coronary revascularization should be as complete as possible. Grafting the left anterior descending coronary artery (LAD) is important since the high portion of the septum, which is almost always functioning, needs to be perfused.

Originally described by Glower and Lowe [1], left ventricular aneurysms are usually associated with single coronary artery disease. The development of collateral circulation is significantly less. As is seen quite commonly in our experience [2, 3], single coronary disease predominates, while in many patients, the infarct-related artery is recanalized, with no significant inducible ischemia in the remote myocardium. These patients benefit from surgical restoration of the adversely remodeled ventricle, as a palliation of their refractory heart failure, if ineligible for cardiac transplantation. In these patients, revascularization has no role.

Some patients have significant disease in two or three coronary arteries, which is associated with inducible ischemia in the remote myocardium requiring surgical revascularization.

Hence, the approach to patients with ischemic cardiomyopathy, with large asynergetic areas of myocardium, will require a three-pronged surgical strategy of restoring ventricle, vessel, and valve.

These patients are in advanced heart failure with large areas of fibrosis and adverse remodeling. Therefore, medical therapy alone is ineffective in reversing adverse remodeling and ameliorating cardiac failure. Faxon et al. demonstrated in the Coronary Artery Surgery Study (CASS) that patients with a LV aneurysm and three-vessel coronary artery disease and patients with clinical heart failure have improved survival with surgical therapy [20].

Intraoperative Anatomy of a Left Ventricular Aneurysm

The anatomy of a typical left ventricular aneurysm has been described by Favoloro et al. [4]. We include this description here to explain the gross pathological appearance of a left ventricular aneurysm.

"From a surgical standpoint, ventricular aneurysm can be defined as a full-thickness scar-tissue replacement of a large segment of the left ventricular wall, usually containing a thrombus and attached to the pericardial sac by adhesions. There was a clear-cut demarcation from the rest of the left ventricle which was easily palpable after the aneurysm was opened.

In anterior aneurysms, the entire anterolateral wall of the left ventricle was replaced by scar tissue with mild to moderate enlargement, increased end-diastolic pressure, and sometimes paradoxical motion. The absence of a frank bulging mass did not exclude a surgical diagnosis of ventricular aneurysm. Resection of the non contractile wall resulted in disappearance of the elevated end-diastolic pressure and clinical improvement.

In a group of patients not included in the series a noncontractile left ventricular wall was demonstrated by cineradiography of the ventricle. Direct observation of the heart in the operative field showed no line of demarcation, and collateral circulation was often recognized on the subepicardial surface. There were definite hypertrophy and dilatation of the wall itself, but myocardial contraction was not effective. Macroscopic evidence of scar tissue was not present. Resection for this type of pathological condition is not indicated. It is our belief that occlusive disease of the coronary circulation can produce myocardial ischemia sufficient to impair muscle contraction but not severe enough to produce necrosis and concomitant scar-tissue replacement. Pathophysiological changes can be reversed in some of these patients by increasing coronary circulation to correct or support the area of perfusion deficit."

Hence, it was evident even in the era prior to nuclear imaging that surgical ventricular restoration had no role in diffusely hypokinetic ventricles with dilatation and areas of viable myocardium. Surgical ventricular restoration has been successful only in ventricles with "large asynergetic areas".[1]

[1]With permission from Favoloro RG et al. Ventricular aneurysm – clinical experience. *The Annals of Thorac Surgery* 1968;6: 227–245.

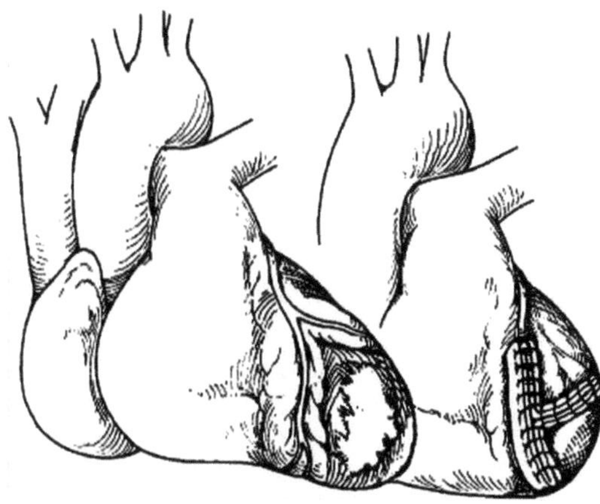

Fig. 6.1 Inverted T closure of left ventricular aneurysm has been done after resection of the aneurysm in an attempt to maintain a more conical shape to the left ventricle. Buttressed sutures are used, and the left anterior descending coronary artery is included in the suture line (With permission from Mills et al. [27]. Copyright Elsevier)

Techniques of Surgical Ventricular Restoration

Aneurysm Resection and Linear Repair

The technique of resection and linear repair was first accomplished in 1955 by Likhoff and Bailey [5]. The surgical procedure of classical linear resection and repair has been detailed by Favoloro et al. [4] (Fig. 6.1).

Ventricular aneurysms are usually associated with pericardial adhesion. Dissection is usually started on total bypass after decompression of the heart. An effort is made to avoid the left phrenic nerve which may be immediately adjacent to the pericardial adhesions. Dissection is done very gently to avoid dislodging mural thrombi. After the left ventricle has been mobilized, the heart is elevated, rotated, and supported with the apex in the uppermost position, a large soft gauze pack placed underneath it. The aneurysm is thus made easily accessible, and since the apex of the heart rests well above the level of the aortic valve, the hazard of air embolization is eliminated. The aneurysm is approached by direct incision in the midportion of the ventricle, and aspiration is applied. If a clot is present, the aorta is totally clamped until it is entirely removed and the left ventricular and atrial chambers have been carefully inspected. The cross-clamp is then released and coronary perfusion reestablished. Direct inspection of the heart usually shows a clear line of demarcation between the fibrous wall of the aneurysm and normal muscle. It is a sound policy to leave a rim of scar tissue at the edges of the resection for support of the sutures. There is a natural fear that complete excision of the aneurysm will compromise left ventricular function by a reduction in the size of its lumen. This is not generally true, and complete excision should be done if restoration of optimum function and effective contraction of the left ventricle are desired. The reconstruction of the left ventricle is done in a linear fashion from base to apex by a continuous running size 0 Mersilene suture, taking full-thickness bites. The initial closure is reinforced by interrupted horizontal size 0 Mersilene sutures which can be placed over Teflon pledgets if there is not enough support at the edges of the resection. Interrupted figure-of-eight 2-0 silk stitches can be used if bleeding points persist in the suture line at the end of reconstruction.

Patient survival improved by this technique of linear plication and excision of the aneurysm, but as the damaged septum was not addressed, retention of this damaged area sometimes led to recurrent heart failure many years later. The septum was addressed in 1978 by Stoney using a flap of scarred tissue [6] (Fig. 6.2), in 1984 by Jatene who imbricated the scar and reformed the elliptical scar [7] (Fig. 6.3), and by Dor in 1984 with exclusion of the scar with endoventricular circular patch plasty (ECVPP) [8] (Fig. 6.4), while ensuring complete revascularization to simultaneously address the ischemic and remote muscle.

Jatene's Technique of Left Ventricular Restoration

The technique adopted by Jatene [9, 10] is briefly discussed below. Most left ventricular aneurysms occur in the anteroseptal region and

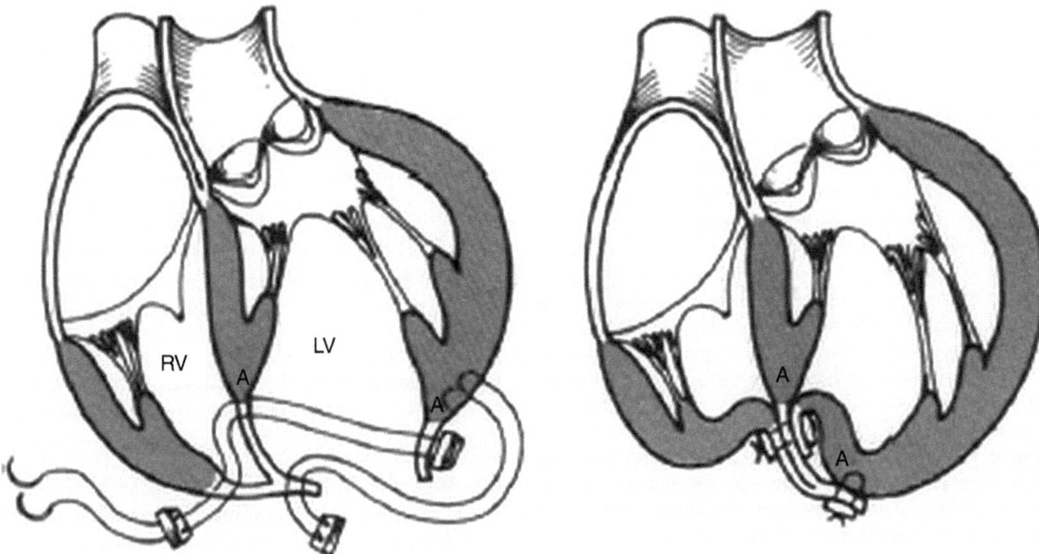

Fig. 6.2 Stoney's repair was used to increase the curvature of the left ventricular segments in a linear repair of the left ventricular aneurysm. The lateral ventricular wall is advanced down the interventricular septum toward the junction of the scar and healthy muscle. *LV* left ventricle, *RV* right ventricle (With permission from Mills et al. [27])

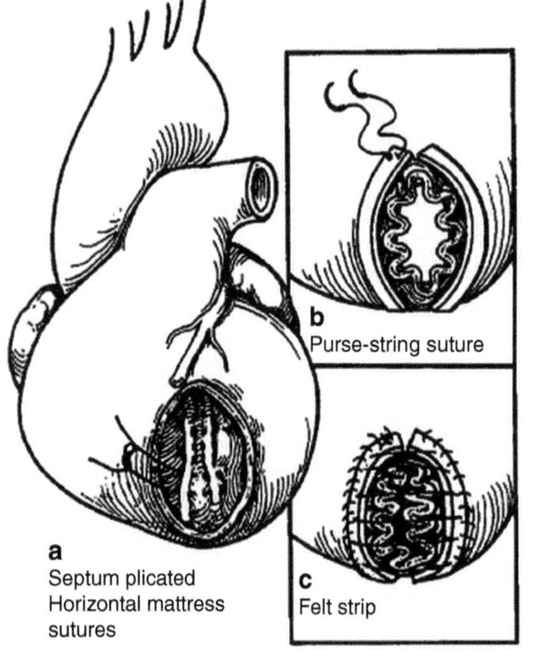

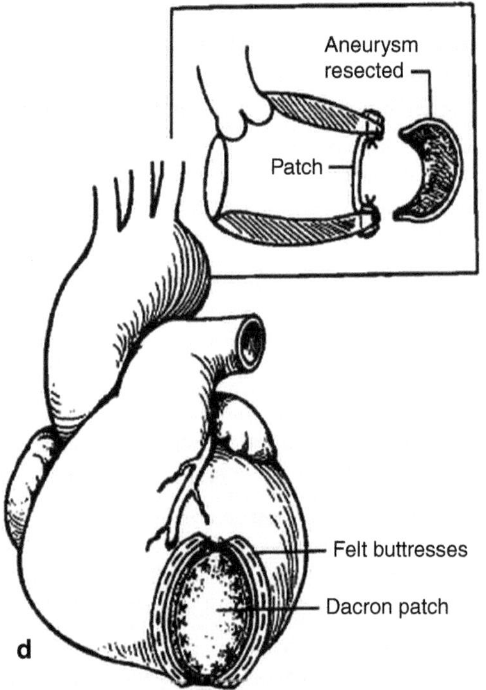

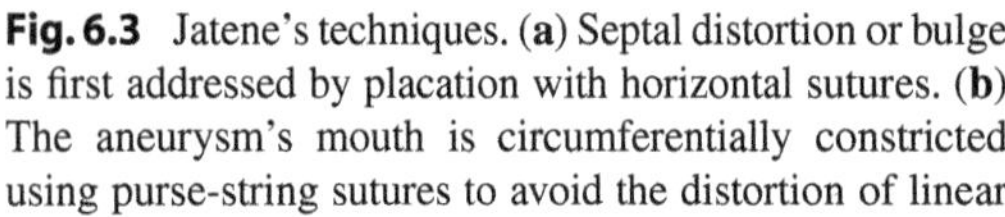

Fig. 6.3 Jatene's techniques. (**a**) Septal distortion or bulge is first addressed by placation with horizontal sutures. (**b**) The aneurysm's mouth is circumferentially constricted using purse-string sutures to avoid the distortion of linear repair. (**c**) Teflon strips sutured to the ventriculotomy site at the apex. (**d**) The intra ventricular Dacron patch with the teflon strips at the ventriculotomy site. (With permission from Mills et al. [27]. Copyright Elsevier)

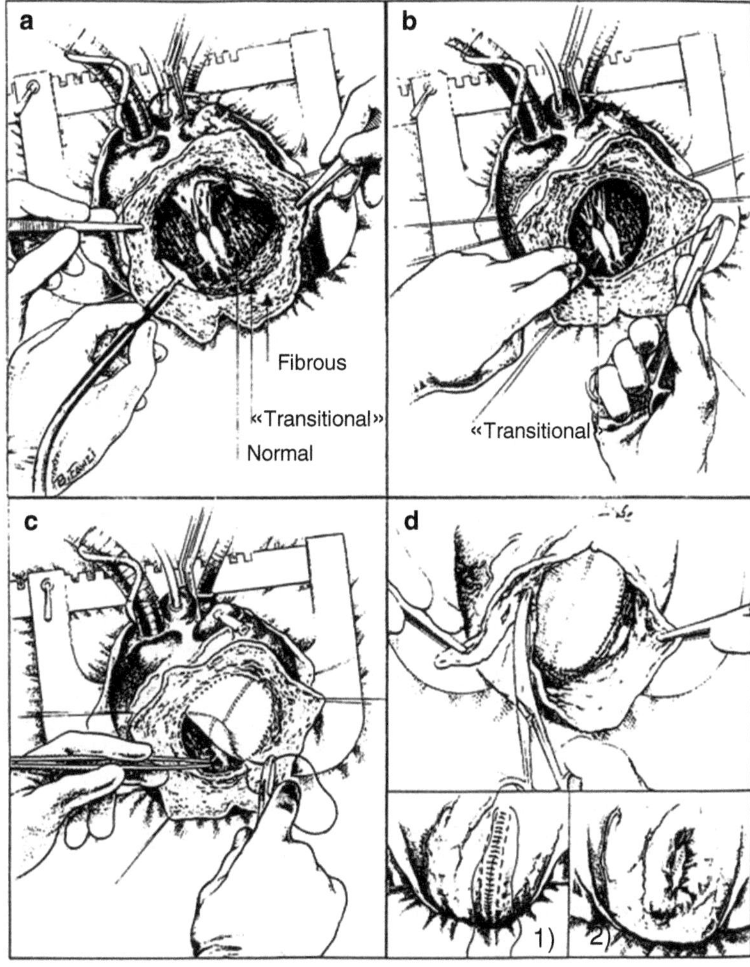

Fig. 6.4 LV remodeling for a large area of scarred postinfarction anterior myocardium. (**a**) The opening of the LV and cryotherapy at the junction between fibrotic and normal endocardium. (**b**) The endoventricular continuous suture with 2-0 monofilament is shown in the intermediate (transitional) zone between normal and totally fibrous tissue to create an artificial neck. Following this, (**c**) shows the Dacron patch anchored with the same 2-0 filament suture. After placement of the EVCPP (**d**), there is resection of exteriorized fibrous tissue and suture (*1*) or folding (*2*) above the patch without stitches. This management of the endoventricular group avoids distortion of the right ventricle (With permission from Dor et al. [23])

involve not only the anterior portion of the free wall of the left ventricle but also the distal ventricular septum. Jatene realized that simple aneurysm resection and linear closure did not correct the septal component of anteroseptal aneurysms and the objective of his new approach was to overcome this deficiency. He did so by introducing the concept of imbricating the involved portion of the septum in order to stabilize it and to give the left ventricular free wall a firm base against which it could contract. Most large anteroseptal aneurysms had dilated bases, and the dilatation of the aneurysm base pulled the non-aneurysmal left ventricular free wall away from the septum. It seemed intuitive that this morphological change in the geometry of the left ventricle would have the effect of decreasing global ventricular function independent of the more direct and apparent adverse effects of the aneurysm. Furthermore, if the base of the resected aneurysm were allowed to persist in its dilated state, the induced dysfunction of the non-aneurysmal left ventricular free wall would continue to exist postoperatively. Jatene's solution was to alleviate that problem by placing an encircling purse-string suture around the base of the aneurysm and tightening it down until the ventricle resumed the shape it would have had if the myocardial infarction had occurred without the complication of an aneurysm. Jatene felt that by reconstructing the normal geometry of the left ventricle as much as possible while removing the aneurysm, the results of surgical therapy should improve. The Jatene technique and the similar technique described by Dor now represent the state-of-the-art in the surgical treatment of left ventricular aneurysms.[2]

Endoventricular Circular Patch Plasty (EVCPP)

This surgical technique [11] was designed to correct not only the visible free-wall component of left ventricular aneurysms but also the septal component which was left unaffected by simple aneurysm resection. In addition, by excluding the involved portion of the septum and placing a "constricting" endocardial patch, a more normal geometry was restored to the left ventricle.

Surgical Technique of EVCPP

Extracorporeal circulation is established, the aorta is cross clamped, and antegrade blood cardioplegia is administered [12]. A left ventricular vent is inserted through the right superior pulmonary vein to provide maximum decompression of the left ventricle. This causes the aneurysmal portion of the left ventricle to collapse, thereby outlining the extent of the aneurysm. The aneurysm is then opened by placing an incision parallel to and 2–3 cm lateral to the left anterior descending coronary artery. The extent of endocardial scarring is determined and the junction between the endocardial scar and normal myocardium is identified throughout the entire circumference of the aneurysm. If the patient has had either spontaneous or inducible ventricular tachycardia preoperatively, a plane of dissection is developed between the endocardial scar covering the distal septum and the underlying septal myocardium. In most cases, this septal scar is resected. In some instances, however, the septal scar is strong enough and the flap is large enough to be used later as an autologous patch for closing the ventricle. In such cases, the base of the flap of septal scar is left in place and the junction of its base with the septum is cryoablated throughout its length. Regardlessofwhetherthisvautologousvflap of scar or a Dacron patch is used to close the ventricle, if the patient has had either spontaneous or inducible ventricular tachycardia, the entire circumference of the nonresected scar is cryoablated. If no ventricular tachycardia is present preoperatively, neither endocardial scar resection nor endocardial cryoablation is used.

A continuous 2-0 monofilament suture is placed around the entire circumference of the base of the aneurysm at the junction of the scar and normal myocardium. This circumferential suture is placed at sufficient depth in the subendocardium to be certain that it will not tear out when tightened. It is placed together with inserting interrupted sutures around this oval orifice to prepare for placing an overlying patch. After inserting these interrupted sutures into suture holders, an operative arrangement is created that mirrors standard surgical methods that are routinely used during valve replacement or repair. Consequently, patch placement now becomes a commonplace surgical procedure, since the only real change relates to how the operator visualizes the goal. Cardiac surgeons are comfortable in placing interrupted or continuous sutures as they surround an aortic or mitral valve orifice during aortic or mitral valve replacement or repair. Consequently, only surgical perspective must change when a patch is used to cover the newly constructed Fontan oval within the ventricle during restoration.

Available methods include direct closure without a patch, folding a septal rim of scar, use of a Dacron patch, autologous pericardium soaked in glutaraldehyde to prevent shrinking, or a commercial bovine pericardial patch with a pericardial rim (like with a valve prosthesis). The suture is tightened so that the dilated base of the aneurysm is narrowed and a more normal shape of the ventricle is attained. There is no absolute formula for how tight to secure this purse-string suture. Rather, the surgeon must envision what the ventricle would look like in the absence of an aneurysm and tighten the suture accordingly. From a practical standpoint, the purse-string suture is usually pulled quite tightly. The degree of tightening of the purse-string suture determines the size of the remaining opening in the ventricle and, therefore, the size of the endocardial patch to be used for closure.

[2]This article was published in Dor et al. [23]. Copyright Elsevier.

Recent modifications of the EVCPP have used an expandable intraventricular sizing balloon of 55 mL/m^2 body surface area, in order to size the restored ventricular cavity and avoid decreasing the cavity too much and thereby prevent postoperative diastolic dysfunction [13].

The patch is usually 2–3 cm in diameter and oval in shape and the material is either Dacron (Hemashield; Meadox Medicals, Inc., Oakland, NJ) or pericardium. If the flap of septal scar is to be used, its size must also conform to that of the ventricular opening after the purse-string has been tightened down. The free edge of the septal scar opposite the septal hinge is modeled in a half-circle of proper size to provide for optimal closure.

If a Dacron patch is used, it is first anchored to the septal side of the opening and then tailored to the proper size for optimal closure of the ventricle. A 2-0 monofilament suture placed in a continuous fashion. Before securing this continuous suture, it is stretched at each point with a small nerve hook to be certain that it is as light as possible. Once the patch has been sutured into position to close the endocardial opening, Resorcine Formol glue (F.I.I., St. Just Malmont, France) is applied to the suture line in a liberal fashion to secure the closure.

If the procedure requires a large portion of the septum to the excluded, it may be difficult or even impossible to reapproximate the superficial tissues external to the patch without leaving an undrained cavity between the reapproximated layer and the endocardial patch. In cases in which a large portion of the ventricular septum has been excluded, the edges of the excluded aneurysm are folded down and attached to the edges of the endocardial patch. This reinforces the suture line, further securing the patch and improving hemostasis.

When less of the septum is excluded and there is sufficient free-wall aneurysmal tissue still attached to the septum, the excluded tissue beyond the level of the endocardial patch may be reapproximated over the endocardial patch. The excess tissue (except for the septum) can also be partially resected, leaving the endocardial patch uncovered. This was the most common closure employed originally (1984–1987) and results in a two-apex ventricle.

Repair of Posterior Aneurysms

Posterior-basilar aneurysms were repaired by opening the ventricle through a longitudinal incision through the aneurysm wall or by detaching the neck of the aneurysm from the posterior left ventricle. If either spontaneous or inducible ventricular tachycardia were present preoperatively, the endocardial scar associated with the aneurysm is mobilized and resected. The left ventricular cavity was reconstructed by anchoring the base of a triangular patch to the external surface of the posterior mitral valve annulus within the left ventricular cavity. The apex of the patch is sutured to the base of the posterior papillary muscle to restore the normal size and shape of the left ventricular cavity.

This surgical technique depended heavily on the identification of the junction between scar and normal myocardium. However, in longstanding ischemic cardiomyopathies, the ventricles were frequently globally dilated with no localized region that was amenable to repair. In addition, the transitional boundary between scar and normal myocardium was not as definitive and easily detected. In such ventricles, the endocardial patch was placed 1–1.5 cm outside the rim of obviously contractile myocardium because in this situation, the only goal that might improve left ventricular function is the reestablishment of a more reasonably sized left ventricular cavity.

On the other hand, if the ventricular aneurysm was very small and well localized, the ventricle was opened through what might appear to be normal muscle adjacent to the ventricle apex. The endocardial scar in such ventricles is usually confined primarily to the most distal septum with slight extension onto to apex. The circumferential subendocardial purse-string suture is, therefore, placed higher up on the septum than on the lateral wall, and thus a "new" ventricular apex is created slightly lateral to the previous apex. The purse-string suture can usually be tightened down to an opening of only 1 cm diameter which can be easily closed with a small pericardial patch.

A total of 34% of patients had a preoperative ejection fraction ≤0.30. The mean preoperative pulmonary artery pressure was ≥25 mmHg in 31% of patients. A Dacron patch was used in 61% of patients, and autologous pericardium or the septal endocardial scar was used as a patch in 39%. Endocardial resection was performed in 40% of patients. Myocardial revascularization was performed in 94.5% of all patients, and at least one internal thoracic artery was employed in 85% of those cases.

The overall operative (30-day) mortality in this series was approximately 7%. As expected, the operative mortality is heavily dependent on the preoperative status of the patient. Preoperative risk factors for an increased operative mortality include refractory heart failure, ischemic ventricular septal defects, refractory ventricular tachycardia, and the need for emergency surgery. In these patients, the operative mortality rate varied between 15% and 20%. For elective surgery in the remainder of patients, the operative mortality was 5%. Early and late hemodynamic evaluation has shown a mean improvement in left ventricular ejection fraction postoperatively of 0.10. In addition to functional improvement, ventricular arrhythmias have been controlled without spontaneous or inducible tachycardia in over 90% of patients.

Modified Linear Repair

Lynda Mickleborough's Technique of Modified Linear Repair

This approach is applicable for all types of aneurysms (broad-based or narrow-necked, true or false). Advantages of this technique are that it is relatively simple, it provides reproducible results, and it can be adapted for a variety of intraoperative situations (calcified or noncalcified ventricular aneurysms) [14]. The only situation in which a more complex type of endoaneurysmorrhaphy repair technique may be advantageous is in cases of acute infarction where friable tissues may make a linear closure difficult or impossible to perform.

Surgical Technique of Modified Linear Repair

Left ventricular aneurysms should be approached through a midline sternotomy [15]. When extensive pericardial adhesions are encountered, mobilization of the heart should be kept to a minimum until cannulation of the aorta and the atrium has been accomplished. Double venous cannulation is recommended for most aneurysm repairs.

After cannulation, adhesions are dissected and the heart is mobilized. (In the case of contained free-wall rupture or "false aneurysm," final dissection into the aneurysmal sac should be delayed until after going on cardiopulmonary bypass.) In many cases, with clear-cut scarring and thinning, the extent of the aneurysm is obvious. In others, inspection reveals an area of mixed scar and viable muscle with no obvious thinning. After placing such patients on cardiopulmonary bypass with decompression of the left ventricle, an area of dimpling or collapse may become obvious. If thinning of the infarct area is not obvious, simple needle aspiration can be used to determine the degree of thinning and the need for resection and repair.

Once the presence of a resectable area of thinned wall has been confirmed, the aneurysm is opened. Stay sutures are applied to the epicardial surface of the scarred area.

In patients with intraventricular clot, the edges of the incision are retracted with clamps and the clot is mobilized and removed in one piece if possible. A flexible sucker is used to decompress and empty the left ventricular cavity while clot is being removed.

Any obvious thinned transmural scar is excised. With the heart open and beating, the surrounding edges are palpated and assessed for contractility. Areas capable of significant contraction or wall thickening in the unloaded state are not resected but revascularized whenever possible, whereas areas that do not contract are considered for excision.

Before final trimming, the size and shape of the remaining left ventricular cavity is evaluated. When the residual chamber is of relatively normal size and shape, linear closure can be easily accomplished. In patients with extensive coro-

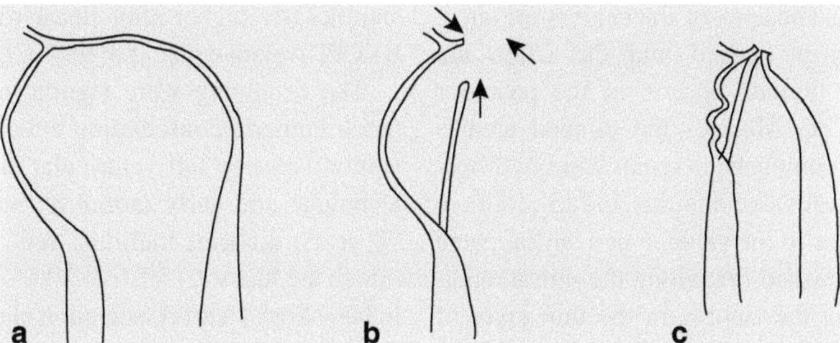

Fig. 6.5 Technique of septal aneurysm patch exclusion. (**a**) Apical aneurysm with significant thinning and aneurysmal involvement of the distal septum. (**b**) Pericardial patch is sewn to preserved normal area of the septum on three sides. (**c**) Patch is pulled tight and the anterior edge incorporated into the modified linear closure effectively excluding the aneurysmal portion of the septum from the residual left ventricle cavity. The (*arrows*) signify the excluded area corresponding to the ventricular aneurysm at the apex (With permission from Mickleborough et al. [47]. Copyright Elsevier)

nary artery disease, marked chamber dilatation, diffuse hypokinesis, and distortion of ventricular shape, it is not possible to restore the ventricular cavity toward normal size or shape with any repair technique (Fig. 6.5). In such patients, for linear closure to be accomplished without distorting left ventricular geometry (specifically the relationship between papillary muscle and the septum), a portion of the nonfunctioning wall may have to be left behind. In these difficult cases, the final resection margins are determined with these considerations in mind.

In patients with marked thinning of the septum or an obvious septal aneurysm, a patch septoplasty should be performed using bovine preserved pericardium. The patch is applied to the left ventricular aspect of the septum and sewn in place to the surrounding normal myocardium on three sides with 4-0 prolene. Anteriorly, the patch is incorporated into the linear ventriculotomy repair.

Aneurysm excision and/or septoplasty are performed on the open beating heart. Using the principles of excision as previously described, in many cases the excised specimen is composed of a mixture of infarcted and viable muscle, and it is not possible to leave behind a rim of fibrous tissue as described in the classic description of aneurysm repair. In such cases, closing sutures have to be placed through fairly thick areas of myocardium. The thinned edges of the aneurysmal sac are retracted with clamps. The limits of the resection margins have been determined by palpation and the thinned noncontractile area is being excised. The incision is closed with mattress sutures of 2-0 prolene buttressed by felt strips. The sutures are placed further apart on the tissue than on the felt so as to plicate the length of the incision in the closure. This technique helps to restore the shape of the ventricle toward normal. Starting at each end, sutures are tied leaving an area for de-airing in the center of the closure. Following aneurysm repair, in those patients requiring aortocoronary bypass grafting, the aorta is cross clamped and cardioplegia is performed using a combination of antegrade and retrograde delivery. Diseased arteries are bypassed whenever possible. The proximal portion of the left anterior descending (LAD) is revascularized even if the distal vessel has been amputated in the repair. Revascularization of even a small part of the septum may be important in improving short- and long-term results in these patients.

In most patients with an inferior aneurysm, the principles of tissue resection and repair are identical to those described for anterior aneurysms. In some cases, however, thin scar extends up to the level of the mitral valve apparatus, and it would be impossible to excise the thinned area and reapproximate the edges without plicating or distorting the valve ring. In these patients, principles of linear closure are modified in the following way: The apex of the heart is elevated. The aneurysm is opened and the edges are retracted. The thinned portion of the posterior wall is indicated. Most of the thinned area is resected. To accomplish the repair without distortion of the mitral valve annulus and to reinforce the closure close to the valve, a pericardial patch is used. It is attached first along the mitral annulus. After tying the sutures in the thin layer of scar, the pericardial patch is reflected posteriorly to cover and reinforce the repair. The patch is attached laterally and medially to relatively normal myocardium. The apex of the patch is incorporated into the posterior linear repair which is accomplished as previously described. In the completed posterior repair, an over and over continuous suture is used to complete the closure and ensure hemostasis.[3]

The Surgical Techniques of Linear Repair or Plication and Endoventricular Patch Plasty and Their Impact on Clinical Outcome

The techniques of surgical ventricular restoration have evolved from the 1950s to now, from simple excision and linear closure to geometric repair with endoventricular patch plasty.

Early and long-term results were compared between the two techniques of surgery by Lundblad et al. [16]. The early mortality (<30 days) was 8.2% (13 patients) for the whole material. Early mortality was 15.4% in the first 39 patients (95% linear repair), 7.5% in the next 40 patients (77.5% linear repair), 2.5% in the following 40 patients (7.5% linear repair), and 7.5% in the last 40 patients (7.5% linear repair). The crude risk of early mortality was significantly higher after linear repair than after EVCPP (OR, 3.8; 95% CI, 1.1–13.4). Overall 5-year cumulative survival was 78% and was significantly higher in the EVCPP group (91.4%) than in the linear repair group (70.1%). The crude risk of total mortality was significantly higher after linear repair than after EVCPP (relative risk, 2.8; 95% CI, 1.3–5.9).

The following were significant confounders (>5% numeric confounding effect) for the association between left ventricular aneurysm repair technique and early mortality: age greater than 70 years, diabetes mellitus, ventricular arrhythmia in the history, LVEF of 30% or less, dyspnea in New York Heart Association class 3 or 4, more than one MI in the history, concomitant CABG, and more than two distal anastomoses performed. The following variables were significant confounders for the association between aneurysm repair technique and total mortality: age greater than 70 years, ventricular arrhythmia in the history, more than one MI in the history, and concomitant CABG. When adjusted for multiple confounders, linear repair was associated with higher early mortality (OR, 4.4; 95% CI, 1.1–17.8) and total mortality (relative risk, 4.5; 95% CI, 2.0–9.7) than EVCPP. EVCPP is a more complex and time-consuming procedure than linear repair, and a cardioplegic heart was often considered to be helpful during patch implantation but not essential in simple linear resection. Accordingly, CPB and aortic cross-clamp times were significantly longer in the EVCPP group. These two variables were not adjusted for in the regression analyses because they are only surrogates for the repair technique. Linear resection dominated early in the series and EVCPP dominated later, but with some overlapping. The effect of learning curve of the institutional team could therefore represent a potential bias in favor of EVCPP. However, the date of the operation could not be adjusted for in the regression analysis because it was highly associated with exposure (repair technique), being a surrogate for the same phenomenon.

Shapira et al. [17] compared the two techniques in a smaller patient group and found similar results (Fig. 6.6). The two groups were matched with respect to age, gender, comorbid risk factors, functional class, urgency of the operation, and concomitant procedures. The duration of cardiopulmonary bypass and aortic cross-clamp time were similar. Concomitant myocardial revascularization was performed in 18 patients

[3]With permission from Mickleborough LL et al. Ventricular reconstruction for ischemic cardiomyopathy. *The Annals of Thoracic Surgery* 2003;75: S6–S12.

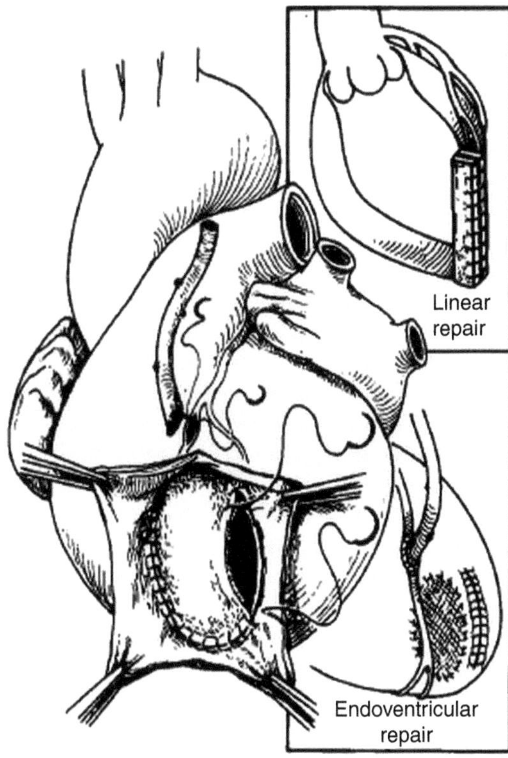

Fig. 6.6 Descriptive comparison of linear plication and repair with endoventricular circular patch plasty (With permission from Mills et al. [27]. Copyright Elsevier)

(90%) with linear repair and 21 patients (78%) with endoaneurysmorrhaphy ($p = 0.18$). The average number of grafts per patient in the linear repair group was 2.5 ± 1.1, and in the endoaneurysmorrhaphy group, it was 2.2 ± 1.0 ($p = 0.39$). Specifically, the left anterior descending coronary artery was grafted in 13 patients (65%) in the linear repair group and 19 patients (70%) in the endoaneurysmorrhaphy group ($p = 0.23$). Thirty-day operative mortality after linear repair was 10%, and after endoaneurysmorrhaphy it was 3.7%, but the difference was too small to reach significance ($p = 0.32$). A greater increase in the early postoperative left ventricular ejection fraction was observed after endoaneurysmorrhaphy: 0.51 ± 0.64 versus 0.18 ± 0.48 ($p = 0.036$). Functional status was significantly better after endoaneurysmorrhaphy than after linear repair: The mean New York Heart Association functional class at the time of follow-up was 1.7 ± 0.9 versus 2.4 ± 1.2 ($p = 0.0001$), and the percentage of patients in New York Heart Association functional class I/II was 88% versus 53% ($p = 0.01$). The trend toward reduced mortality (3.7% vs. 10%) and reduced use of intra-aortic balloon pumps (3.7% vs. 15%) after endoaneurysmorrhaphy did not reach significance presumably because of the small sample size.

Ventricular Arrhythmias and Surgical Technique

Ventricular arrhythmia arises in the border zone between viable and dead myocardium, usually on the interventricular septum. Simple linear resection with or without concomitant CABG often fails to control ventricular arrhythmia. EVCPP and linear resection combined with septoplasty might reduce wall tension on the septal border zone, and it is hypothesized that this might have an inherent antiarrhythmic effect.

Revascularization and Ventricular Restoration

Concomitant CABG is highly recommended for two reasons. First, it reduces or prevents angina pectoris. Second, although the LAD is occluded and the periphery on the free wall is thin or calcified, an internal mammary graft to the LAD might be particularly important to improve septal perfusion and control ventricular arrhythmia. In the present study, revascularization of the LAD was significantly more frequent in the EVCPP group (72%) than in the linear repair group (39%). The importance of an internal mammary graft to the LAD during complex operations was probably underestimated in the first period of the series, when linear repair dominated. Moreover, with this technique, the aneurysmal sac is partly removed, and the remnant is used for closure of the LV, which could render revascularization of the LAD more difficult. During EVCPP, more of the aneurysmal sac is retained, and therefore the conditions for revascularization of the LAD might be better.

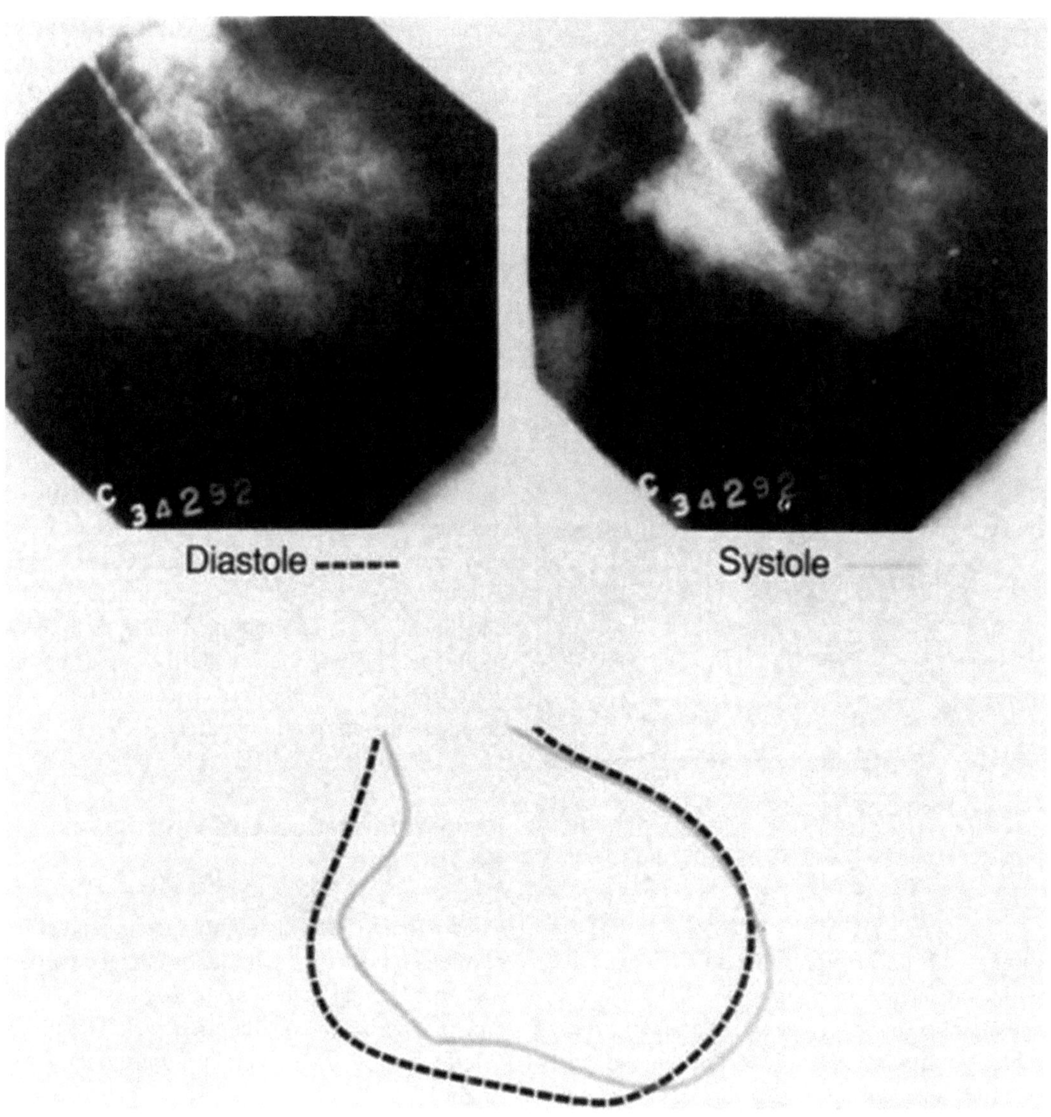

Fig. 6.7 Representative diastolic and systolic frames from ventriculogram of patient in this series. Ventricular wall is diffusely hypokinetic. Chamber is markedly dilated and distorted (With permission from Mickleborough et al. [14]. Copyright Elsevier)

Left Ventricular Function and Surgical Technique

EVCPP was introduced as a more physiological repair than the traditional simple linear resection technique. EVCPP is supposed to provide a more physiological apex, whereas the distal end of the LV is more flattened after simple linear repair. EVCPP can improve left ventricular function and is probably more effective than traditional simple linear resection. The present study compares EVCPP with the traditional simple linear resection. The more sophisticated technique of Mickleborough and associates, using septoplasty and linear repair, might provide equally good results as EVCPP (Fig. 6.7).

Shapira's study also confirms previous reports that repair of left ventricular aneurysm using "plastic" reconstructive techniques (such as endoaneurysmorrhaphy) results in a significantly greater postoperative increase in left ventricular ejection fraction as compared with linear repair. Although both methods eliminate the paradoxical motion of the left ventricular free wall, endoaneurysmorrhaphy also excludes the septal akinesis and theoretically may decrease the tension on the transitional zone, encourage revascularization of the left anterior descending artery, and improve the alignment of the muscle fibers, resulting in a more physiological contraction. The long-term results of better functional class with EVCPP are demonstrated in this study, which may actually reflect better restored ventricular geometry and revascularization.

Due to these and several other smaller series demonstrating conflicting reports, Parolari et al. [18] conducted a meta-analysis of 18 non-randomized studies comparing linear repair and EVCPP. Since meta-analysis may provide additional statistical power that overcomes the limited sample size of most studies together with the low incidence of the major end points, for example, in-hospital mortality, this study was conducted as a retrospective analysis. Eighteen trials were identified and included in the analysis with a total of 1,814 and 803 patients who underwent linear and geometric reconstruction, respectively. The analysis showed a significantly increased risk of in-hospital death for patients undergoing linear reconstruction (RR = 1.59, 95% CI: 1.12–2.26, $p=0.01$). The temporal sequence of surgical procedure was found of particular relevance, when separate analyses were performed on studies where both techniques were used in temporal sequence and on studies where both techniques were used simultaneously. The subanalysis of studies in which linear reconstruction was adopted mainly in the first period of time, and geometric reconstruction was adopted in a later phase, still showed a significant advantage in terms of in-hospital mortality for patients undergoing geometric reconstruction ($n=11$ studies, RR = 1.89, 95% CI: 1.22–2.93, $p=0.004$). By contrast, when the two surgical approaches were carried out in the same time lag, there was no difference between linear and geometric reconstruction techniques in terms of in-hospital mortality ($n=7$ studies, RR = 1.04, 95% CI: 0.57–1.92, $p=0.89$). Interestingly, this analysis showed that, with current literature evidence, it is not possible to document differences between these two strategies for three of the major complications occurring after cardiac surgical procedures: perioperative myocardial infarction, stroke, and renal failure.

The findings of this meta-analysis must be interpreted with some caution. First, the design of the study may lack the experimental element of a random allocation to the linear or to the geometric reconstruction techniques, and very few studies included in the meta-analysis reported the criteria considered by the individual surgeons to allocate patients to either group. It is well known that meta-analysis is most effective when analyzing randomized studies, but in this case only observational studies were available. Second, the two groups were not comparable for all the factors that can alter the outcome of interest, and confounding factors cannot be excluded.

Another retrospective meta-analysis by Patrick Klein et al. [19] of 62 studies of 12,331 patients showed a weighted average early mortality of 6.9%. This compared favorably to the natural history of LV aneurysms with a reported 5-year survival of 12–47%. Cumulative 1-, 5-, and 10-year survival were 88.5%, 71.5%, and 53.9%, respectively. Endoventricular reconstruction showed a reduced risk for both early (RR = 0.79, $p<0.005$) and late (RR = 0.67, $p<0.001$) mortality compared to the linear repair (early: RR = 1.38, $p<0.001$; late: RR = 1.83, $p<0.001$). Early mortality and late mortality were mainly cardiac in origin, with heart failure as predominant cause in respectively 49.7% and 34.5% of the cases. Ventricular arrhythmias caused 16.6% of early deaths and 17.2% of late deaths. Concomitant CABG significantly decreased late mortality (RR = 0.28, $p<0.001$) without increasing early mortality (RR = 1.018, $p=0.858$). Concomitant mitral valve surgery showed both an increased risk for early (RR = 1.57, $p=0.001$) and late mortality (RR = 4.28, $p<0.001$). No clinical or hemodynamic parameters were found to influence mortality. It is noteworthy that only one-third of patients included in the current analysis were operated for heart failure (14 studies, 4,135 patients).

The linear repair technique cannot exclude the septal scar and also carries the risk of creating a restrictive residual LV cavity, especially in large aneurysms, leading to diastolic dysfunction and LV failure [21–23]. Sizing of the residual LV cavity in EVCPP, either by an intracavitary balloon or a commercially available shaper device to a volume of 50–60 mL/m^2 BSA, avoids creating a residual LV cavity that is restrictive [24–26]. Because of the limited number of patients in the currently available reports, the relative risks for early mortality calculated for the linear repair with septoplasty, and the septoexclusion techniques did not reach statistical significance. Possibly, the complete exclusion of the septal scar and the more anatomical reconstruction with EVCPP led to a more efficient myocardial fiber orientation and systolic function contributing to this reduction in late mortality [13, 24]. Also, the fact that grafting the left anterior descending coronary artery is more feasible in the EVCPP technique may play a role [16, 27].

With respect to the technique of reconstructing the LV cavity, three possible explanations exist for early and late LV failure: first, the aforementioned problem of creating a restrictive residual LV cavity, leading to diastolic dysfunction and LV failure; second, leaving a too large residual LV cavity only partially reverses the remodeling process and may lead to redilatation of the left ventricle. Also, a residual large akinetic area has been mentioned as possible cause for redilatation. Ueno et al. demonstrated redilatation and increasing sphericity after Dor and SAVE procedures at intermediate follow-up, resulting in increased wall tension with reduced compliance as possible causes for late heart failure [28]. Raman et al. associated the use of a stiff and relatively big patch in EVCPP as cause for some adverse long-term outcomes [29]. Patch size, shape, and orientation may prove to be important in preventing adverse ventricular remodeling over time, as Cirillo et al. have shown in a small group with an EVCPP technique using a small, obliquely oriented, and oval-shaped patch [30]. Third, insufficient residual remote myocardium to survive the procedure and to translate the surgically induced morphological changes to functional improvement leads to LV failure.

Ventricular Arrhythmias

Late ventricular arrhythmias have been related to ventricular dilatation with high wall stress and stretch [31]. It has been postulated that LV reconstruction surgery due to volume reduction reduces arrhythmogenicity. Exclusion of the myocardial scar, concomitant complete revascularization, and mechanical resynchronization further reduces the trigger for electrical instability and may render the need for an implantable cardioverter-defibrillator (ICD) unnecessary [31, 32]. Some authors like Dor et al. [23] and Mickleborough et al. [33] advocate routine use of concomitant endocardiectomy of the border zone of viable and nonviable myocardium and cryotherapy to further decrease the risk of ventricular arrhythmias. These authors have reported a low late incidence of ventricular arrhythmias with this strategy. The relatively high incidence of death due to ventricular arrhythmias observed in the present pooled analysis raises the question whether LV reshaping with volume reduction, scar exclusion, and revascularization is sufficiently anti-arrhythmogenic to make adjunctive device therapy of little use.

Effect of Concomitant Procedures on Mortality

The concomitant myocardial revascularization with LV reconstruction surgery improved late survival without increasing the risk for early mortality. Besides symptomatic relief of angina, revascularization of viable, remote myocardium in non-scarred segments may improve compensatory contractile function [34]. Also, revascularization of the proximal left anterior descending coronary artery to improve septal perfusion may contribute favorably [16]. Another contributing factor could be that revascularization further reduced the risk for late ventricular arrhythmias. These factors probably outweigh the increase in operative and extracorporeal circulation time and thus did not result in higher early mortality. This finding underlines the importance of (complete) revascularization in these patients.

Mitral Valve Surgery

In patients with previous anterior myocardial infarction, functional mitral regurgitation occurs mainly in the setting of LV dilatation, with tethering of the mitral valve leaflets, displacement of the subvalvular apparatus, and dilatation of the mitral annulus causing secondary incompetence of the mitral valve. Functional mitral regurgitation therefore mainly reflects a more advanced stage of disease, and has been shown to be associated with an increased mortality, independent of the degree of underlying LV dysfunction [35–37]. The need for mitral valve surgery in LV reconstruction surgery is therefore an index of gravity. This is by no means an argument not to perform mitral valve surgery in these patients, since mitral regurgitation-related volume overload has been shown to promote further LV remodeling and progression of heart failure. Correcting mitral regurgitation improves clinical functional class and may prevent LV redilatation [26]. However, this analysis does not permit any conclusion on the benefits of mitral valve surgery, since no comparison between treated and nontreated patients was available in the literature.

The failure of LVEF, LV volumes, age, gender, and time interval post-myocardial infarction in predicting outcome questions the use of these parameters in risk stratification for these patients. Newer models using advanced imaging techniques that can test for the functional capacity of the remote myocardium, like (contrast-enhanced) magnetic resonance imaging or (3D) echocardiographically derived wall motion score indexes, may prove useful for improved risk stratification.

Vural et al. [38] also compared the two techniques of left ventricular reconstruction done at their center. However, this comparison was offset by a major limitation of the preoperative cardiac states of the two repair groups (circular and linear) not being identical. Generally, the choice for the repair technique was not made randomly, but rather it depended on factors such as size and extension of the scarred tissue. An extensive and definite fibrotic aneurysmal sac with a well-formed neck generally led the surgeon to the circular repair; while in a small wide-based aneurysm vaguely separated from the surrounding viable myocardium, a small plication was usually preferred. In cases with extensive septal involvement, either septal plication was added to the linear repair or patch endoaneurysmorrhaphy was employed. The repair method (endoaneurysmorrhaphy vs. linear) did not influence early mortality or survival; further, there was no evidence for any superiority of circular repair on immediate cardiac performance, by means of low cardiac output development. But among the survivors, most patients in class I were the patients who had undergone circular repair. Thus, it could be concluded that circular repair may bring some advantages, such as better functional capacity when late results were considered, despite the worse preoperative cardiac condition. Thus, better outcome was expected in the linear closure group which consisted of patients with smaller aneurysms and better myocardial reserve than those in the circular group. In contrast, although the two repair groups were not identical, a more favorable functional status was obtained in the circular closure group, possibly accentuating the advantage of this type of repair.

Modifications of the EVCPP

If the residual ventricular volume is too small, the results will be catastrophic, resulting in the physiology of a restrictive cardiomyopathy. This risk is particularly great if the preoperative chamber is only moderately dilated. If the residual chamber is too large, the benefit will be limited. Menicanti et al. [13] have modified the classical EVCPP due to various drawbacks of the original technique (Fig. 6.8).

To diminish the risk of too large or too small a size of the residual ventricular chamber, Dor introduced the use of an intraventricular balloon filled to a known volume of 60 mL/m^2, to guide the restoration and to leave an adequate residual chamber. The volume 60 mL/m^2 was chosen after study of postoperative angiograms. This value may be too small if the preoperative volume is very large; thus, when preoperative volumes are greater than 150 mL/m^2, 15% is added to the volume of the balloon (approximately 70 mL/m^2).

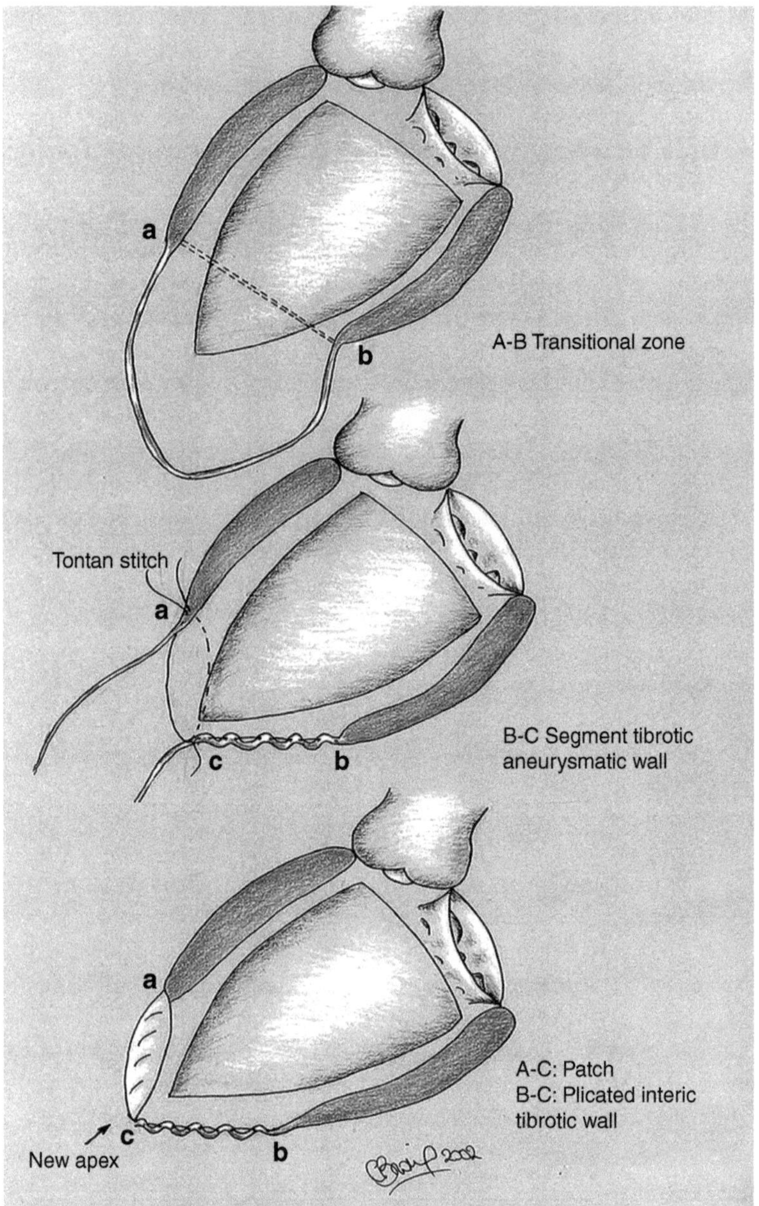

Fig. 6.8 Menicanti's modification of Dor's endoventricular circular patch plasty (With permission from Menicanti and Di Donato [13]. Copyright Elsevier)

The opening of the ventricle is closed with a Dacron patch if the diameter is 3 cm or greater. If it is smaller than 3 cm, the closure is performed with simple stitches tangential to the balloon. In this case, a second stratum with the excluded tissue is sutured on the first suture to avoid bleeding. If the closure is done by patch, few millimeters of external borders is left in the everting way so that it is easy to add stitches for good hemostasis, if needed.

Predictors of Adverse Outcomes After Surgical Ventricular Restoration

The severity of LV remodeling is based on LV shape rather than volume and ejection fraction (EF). Marco Pocar [39] in his study identified baseline mitral regurgitation and sphericity index as independent predictors of recurrent heart failure ($p=0.025$; HR = 7.80 (95% CIs: 1.29–47.19)) and LV re-remodeling ($p = 0.047$; HR = 2.84 (95% CIs: 1.01–7.95)), respectively. When LV redilatation was analyzed, considering the 50 mL/m^2 ESVI threshold as adverse event, both MR and SI were independently predictive ($p = 0.049$; HR = 4.98 (95% CIs: 1.01–24.67) for MR; $p = 0.025$; HR = 6.55 (95% CIs: 1.27–33.86) for SI). Similarly, the probability of recurrent HF or of a 25% increased ESVI at Kaplan–Meier analysis was respectively higher among patients with baseline 2+ MR ($p = 0.008$) and SI ≥0.75 ($p = 0.039$), whereas both predictors generated significantly divergent curves when analyzing the occurrence of a late ESVI ≥50 mL/m^2 ($p = 0.008$ for MR; $p = 0.031$ for SI).

A baseline SI <0.75 showed a much lower probability of late LV re-remodeling and never showed a late ESVI ≥50 mL/m^2. The increased risk of redilatation in case of a more spherical LV before SVR was not surprising because a higher SI is per se expression of a more remodeled LV. In fact, although a proposed conicity index may better reflect regional anteroapical remodeling [40], this applies essentially to the earlier phases that follow anterior myocardial infarction, where the LV silhouette is still deformed by the neck of an aneurysmal sac.

The probability of recurrent heart failure was independently affected by preoperative 2+ MR versus 1+ MR. Similarly, a late postoperative ESVI ≥50 mL/m^2, that is, late SVR failure, could be predicted by 2+ MR. A possible direct benefit on LV function determined by the reshaping of the LV base that follows undersized annuloplasty has been investigated in the experimental setting also, in the absence of significant MR.

Although HF is reversed by the Dor procedure, the latter produces a less elliptical neo-LV compared with its modified approaches aimed at the creation of a longer and more conical LV cavity, with or without implantation of a patch. These findings suggest that the specific benefits of surgical techniques aimed at rebuilding a more conical LV cavity may be more evident in patients with advanced LV remodeling.

In a special report by Gerald Buckberg et al. [41], on Scientific Priorities and Strategic Planning for Development of New Views of Disease, a joint recommendation was finalized with respect to advancement in surgical techniques for SVR. The centerpiece of techniques in surgical heart failure therapy focuses on the application of Laplace's law to justify reduction of LV wall tension through the reduction of its radius of curvature. However, a critical dilemma for these surgical treatments is the final form that the LV volume attains. Should we, for example, remodel a dilated sphere-like LV to a smaller sphere or to a smaller volume that has an ellipsoidal shape? Following the latter course will change fiber orientation and produce an anisotropic and thus heterogeneous structure, which might have a crucial impact on restoring the mechanical and hemodynamic functions of the failing spherical heart toward those of a more normal conical heart.

Hence, several cardiac surgeons like Calafiore et al. [42], Suma et al. [43], Cooley [44], and Parachuri [2, 3] improvised on the technique of SVR with the use of longer endoventricular patches. Ueno has used a modified surgical technique of SVR, the overlapping technique, and demonstrated superior results with respect to ventricular geometry and absence of re-remodeling at midterm when compared with the classical Dor and SAVE techniques [28] (Fig. 6.9).

Cooley has used a variety of other techniques to repair ventricular aneurysms, including plication, septoplasty with plication, patches, septal patches, and overlapping and felt buttresses (Figs. 6.9, 6.10, and 6.11). In 1988, a new method of repair was tried by Cooley and coworkers in a few patients whose ventricular aneurysms were so large that repair by excision would have left too little normal myocardium to restore ventricular function. This technique of intracavitary repair was accomplished with an oval endoventricular patch which was preformed to the ventricular cavity.

Surgical Technique of Cooley's Modification of Endoventricular Aneurysmorrhaphy

A standard median sternotomy incision to expose the heart. The ascending aorta is cannulated for arterial inflow, and the right atrium is

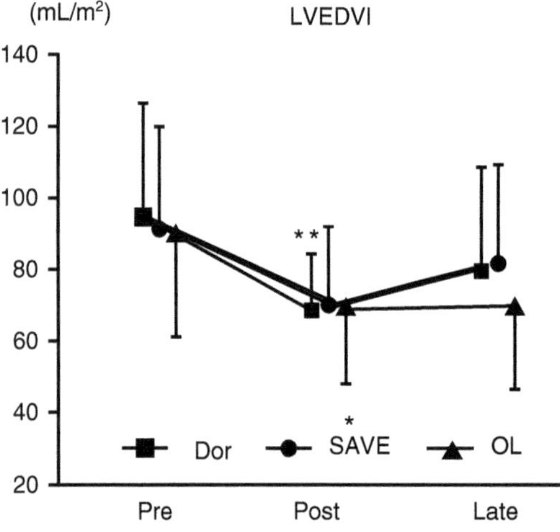

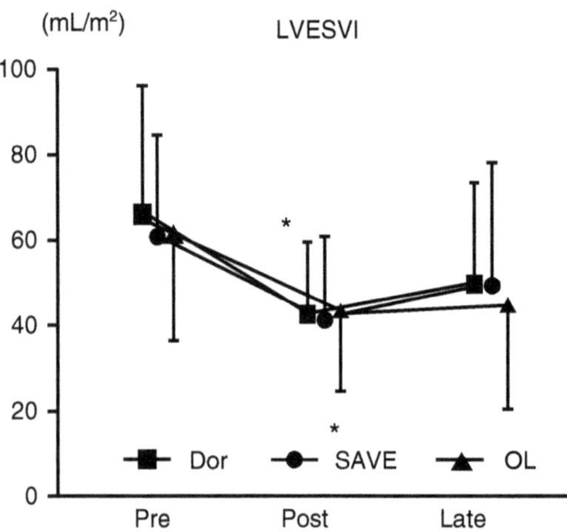

Fig. 6.9 The LVEDVI and LVESVI were significantly reduced immediately after the operation in the Dor and overlapping groups. However, they increased again in the Dor group but remained almost unchanged in the overlapping group at intermediate postoperative follow-up (*LVEDVI* left ventricular end-diastolic volume index, *LVESVI* left ventricular end-systolic volume index, (*) $p<0.05$, (**) $p<0.01$) (With permission from Ueno et al. [28]. Copyright Elsevier)

cannulated for venous return. Moderate general body hypothermia is induced at 28–32°C, after which the heart is arrested by using 500 mL of a 4°C crystalloid solution, which contains 20 mEq of potassium chloride.

The epicardial surface of the left ventricle is dissected from any pericardial adhesions. A longitudinal incision is made over the apex and the thinnest portion of the aneurysm, parallel to the interventricular groove. After the aneurysmal cavity is opened, any thrombus, which is found in about 50% of patients, should be removed. Blood is then evacuated from the ventricle, which makes identifying the extent of fibrosis easier. A transition zone will be apparent between the more normal, maroon-colored myocardium and the whitish, fibrous area of scar tissue.

Once the defect is identified, the surgeon should determine the optimal size and shape of the patch needed to restore the normal geometric dimensions and volume to the ventricle. An elliptical patch of woven Dacron is then tailored to fit the defect. The patch is secured by 2-0 or 3-0 continuous polypropylene sutures into the firm, fibrous tissue.

Although some other surgeons use pericardial patches preserved in glutaraldehyde, the use of a Dacron patch is preferred unless the aneurysm is very large.

Finally, the ventriculotomy is repaired by using continuous 2-0 or 3-0 suture. In making the repair, it is important to avoid crossing the interventricular groove and the left anterior descending coronary artery, even when the artery is diseased or occluded. In most patients, the arterial occlusion was bypassed with an internal mammary artery.

If coronary artery bypass is indicated, it is performed after the aneurysm is repaired, either with an internal mammary artery pedicle or a saphenous vein graft. In any case, complete revascularization should always be performed. Evert in the presence of septal wall dysfunction, the left anterior descending and diagonal arteries should be bypassed.

"Reprinted with permission. Copyright 1981, Texas Heart Institute, Houston. Reddy et al. [48]".

The incidence of developing arrhythmias postoperatively was less in patients who had undergone endoaneurysmorrhaphy than in patients who had linear repair of their aneurysms. Most likely, the arrhythmogenic focus was removed or interrupted when sutures were placed in the aneurysmal border zone. Restoring more normal ventricular geometry reduces myocardial wall stress, which may also change the conduction pattern and, subsequently, decrease the incidence of arrhythmias.

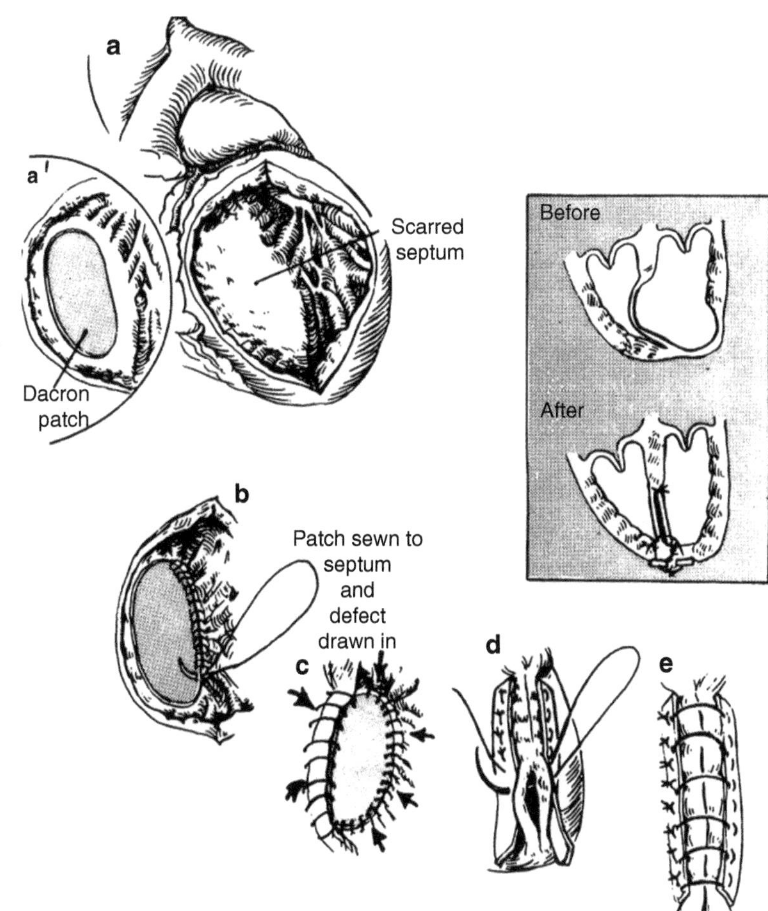

Fig. 6.10 Modified endoventricular repair of left ventricular aneurysm. (**a**) Denotes the scarred septum with the intra ventricular dacron patch sutured to exclude it. (**b**) Depicts suturing of the intra ventricular dacron patch. (**c**) Patch sewn to septum and defect drawn in. (**d**) The ventriculotomy being sutured with two teflon strips on either side. (**e**) Completed closure of the ventriculotomy (With permission from Mills et al. [27]. Copyright Elsevier)

Occasionally, when arrhythmias are a primary indication for surgery, cryoablation, subendocardial resection, or encircling ventriculotomy should be considered in addition to endoaneurysmorrhaphy, especially when the arrhythmogenic focus is in an area that may continue to cause life-threatening arrhythmias after surgery. Two main parameters of left ventricular function improved significantly: mean ejection fraction and New York Heart Association (NYHA) functional class. Actuarial survival rates (including early deaths) were 80.3% at 1 year, 77.6% at 2 years, 76.3% at 3 years, and 68% at 5 years. The predictors of early postoperative mortality were acute myocardial infarction (odds ratio, 6.9; $p<0.0001$), previous cardiac surgery (odds ratio, 3.4; $p<0.0049$), and advanced age (≥70 years) (odds ratio, 3.4; $p<0.0002$). Decreased long-term survival could be predicted by poor ejection fraction (≤30%) (odds ratio, 2.3; $p<0.0066$), NYHA functional class IV status (odds ratio, 2.2; $p<0.0049$), and advanced age (≥70 years) (odds ratio, 2.5; $p<0.0004$). Their results with intracavitary repair of LV aneurysm indicate that this technique, which restores the natural left ventricular geometry, is associated with significant improvement in left ventricular function. Furthermore, despite increased early postoperative mortality in the high-risk patients, there is no significant difference in long-term survival among the survivors of surgery, whether patients are in the lower-risk or the high-risk group.

Although the high-risk patients had an expectedly higher early mortality rate, many of these patients' aneurysms would have been considered inoperable if the traditional linear repair was the only option. Included among these patients who underwent intracavitary repair

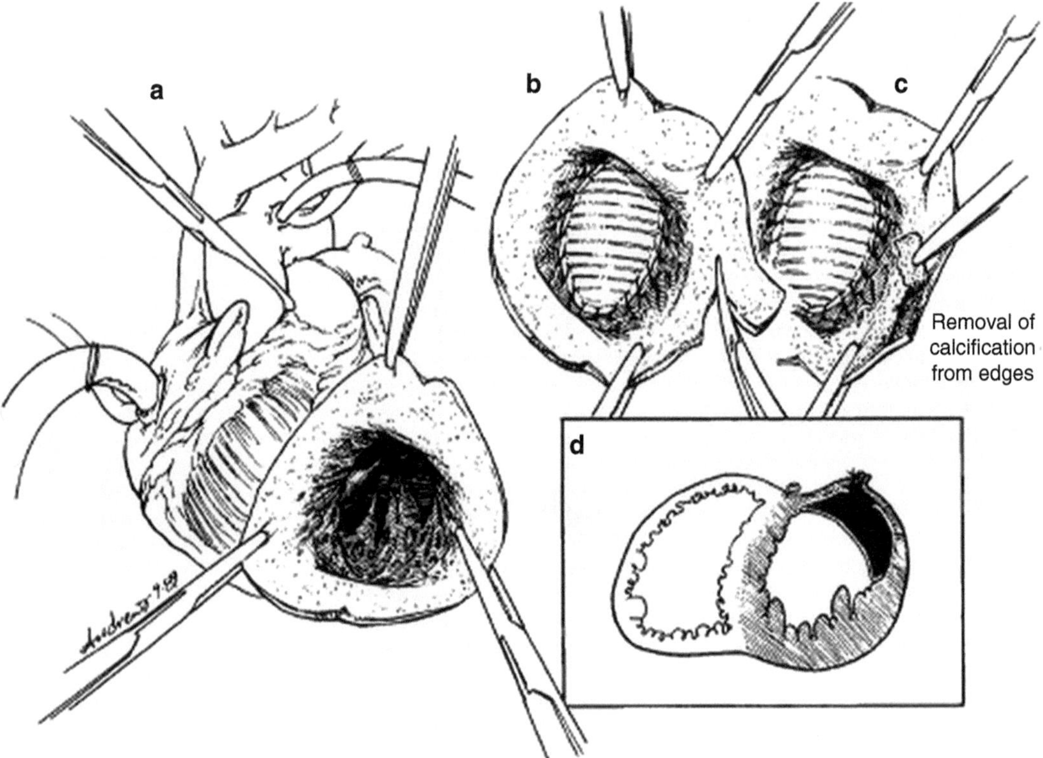

Fig. 6.11 (**a**) Following ventriculotomy, inspection of the ventricular cavity for thombus and calcium. (**b**) and (**c**) removal of calcium and aneurismal exclusion by intraventricular ellipsoid patch. (**d**) Final linear repair over the intraventricular patch plasty (With permission from Mills et al. [27]. Copyright Elsevier)

were many with diffuse left ventricular dilation and densely calcified lesions. In both high- and lower-risk patients, left ventricular function improved, as measured by ejection fraction and by NYHA functional class. When linear and intracavitary repair were compared, it was found that only 51% of patients who underwent linear repair improved after their operations, whereas 76% of those patients who underwent intracavitary repair improved. When ventricular geometry is restored, paradoxical contractile forces and end-diastolic volume both decrease, which, along with increased perfusion from bypass grafting, could account for the improved left ventricular function seen in patients who undergo intracavitary repair.

The Dor technique is addressed to the recovery of a predictable volume but not to the rebuilding of a physiological conical shape. Another French surgeon, Daniel Guilmet, described in the 1980s a technique (overcoat technique) that led to a conical shape of the heart [45]. Calafiore et al. [42] revisited the original Guilmet technique at the end of the 1990s, using some modifications but maintaining the concept. In 2002, they applied, in all patients, techniques finalized to recover a conical shape, septal reshaping [6], evolution of the Guilmet technique, and the Dor operation only in the presence of septoapical scars.

Surgical Technique of Guilmet Procedure

The modified Guilmet procedure(S) included a suture of the scarred anterior wall to the scarred septum with interrupted U sutures. Septal reshaping was used when the septum was more involved than the anterior wall. In this procedure, the length of the patch depends on the distance between the

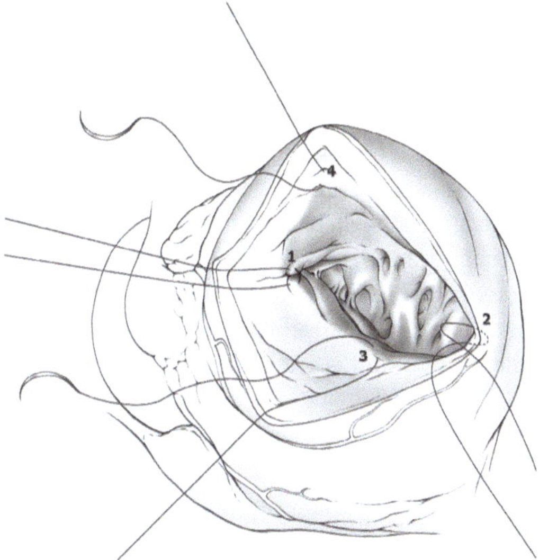

Fig. 6.12 Four stitches are positioned, in the septum at the end of the last interrupted suture (*1*), at the level of the new apex (*2*), deep in the septum (*3*), at the border between the scar and the healthy posterior septum, and in the anterior wall, again at the limit of the scar (*4*) (With permission from Calafiore et al. Elsevier)

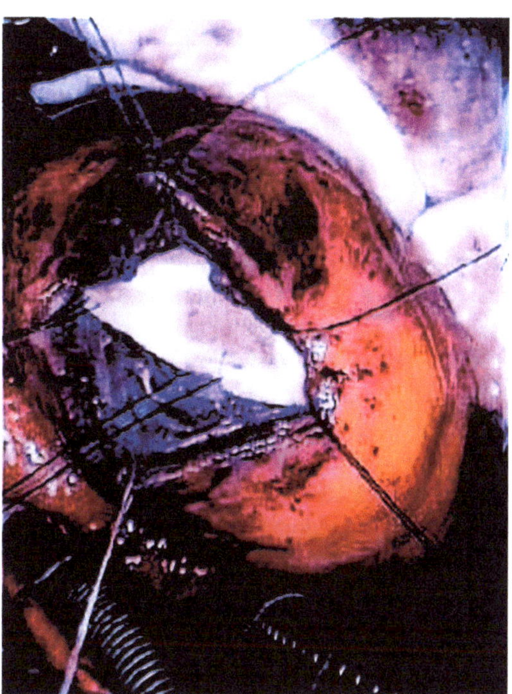

Fig. 6.13 Intraoperative view. An oval dacron patch is tailored and fixed with the four stitches previously placed (With permission from Calafiore et al. [49]. Copyright Elsevier)

highest point and the new apex; its height is related to the LV diastolic volume. If less than 80 mL/m^2, the length/height ratio is 2:1; if 80 mL/m^2 or greater, the ratio was 3:1; and in case of restrictive diastolic dysfunction, the ratio was 3:1 as well. To be sure that the longitudinal diameter was long enough, the position of the new apex had to be roughly 5 cm from the base of the papillary muscles and, for this purpose, could be positioned in the apical scar. The septoapical Dor procedure(V) was used only in case of scars that involved the distal portion of the septum and the apex. Again, the purse-string was positioned roughly 5 cm from the base of the papillary muscles. Mitral valve surgery was performed in patients with septoapical shaping more than in patients subjected to only septal shaping (Figs. 6.12, 6.13, and 6.14).

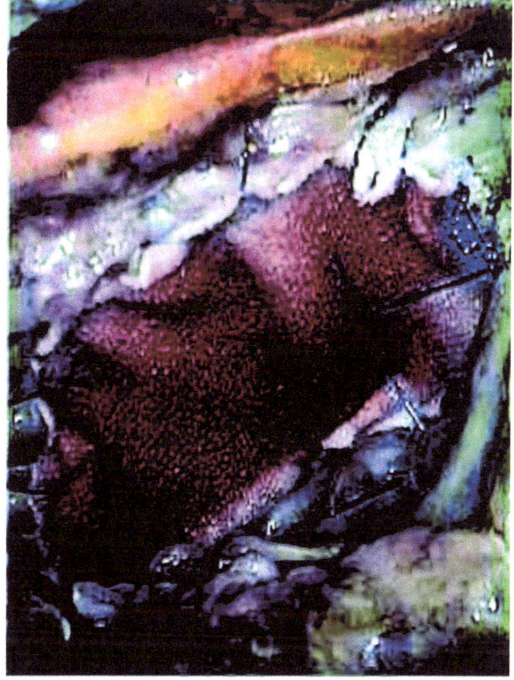

Fig. 6.14 Intraoperative view. The patch is sutured among the septum, the anterior wall, and the new apex (With permission from Calafiore et al. [49]. Copyright Elsevier)

Mortality Benefit

Five-year freedom from death of any cause was 72.9% ± 4.3% in group V versus 81.0% ± 2.9% in group S ($p=0.140$), freedom from cardiac death was 76.3% ± 4.1% versus 86.6% ± 2.6% ($p=0.032$), freedom from any cardiac event was 63.9%±4.7% versus 77.9%±3.3% (p=0.011). After a mean follow-up of 46±43 months, 28 in group V and 30 in group S died of cardiac causes and in 44 cases and 14 cases of noncardiac causes.

Hospitalization for heart failure occurred in 48 patients (19 in group S and 29 in group V). Cox analysis, adjusted for propensity score, showed that the choice of volume rather than shape was a risk factor for late death of any cause, cardiac death, a cardiac event, and any event. Excluding first-month events, freedom from death of any cause was 84.2% (82.1% in group V vs. 86.2% in group S, p=0.0528), freedom from cardiac death was 87.9% (85.1%in group V vs. 90.2%in group S, p <0.003), freedom from cardiac events was 77.1% (71.2% in group V vs. 81.1% in group S, p=0.039), and freedom from any event was 77.1% (69.5% in group V vs. 77.4% in group S, p=0.0211). Cox analysis, adjusted for age, EF, and mitral valve surgery, confirmed that the choice of volume rather than the shape was a risk factor for freedom from cardiac events (hazard ratio, 2.2; 95% CI, 1.2±3.8; p=0.007).

The patients in NYHA class I or II were 77.6% in group V and 89.1% in group. LV reshaping rather than volume reduction was associated with NYHA class improving across time (βcoefficient, 0.82±0.25; p=0.001); patients with lower preoperative NYHA class showed higher probability to remain unchanged or improved (0.34±0.13, p=0.007).

The choice of ventricular shaping and lower preoperative LVEF was found to be associated with EF improving across time. No factors were found to be associated with LV volume increase, sphericity index improvement, and MR impairment across time.

The need for a more physiological shape goes together with the changing pattern of septoapical scars. In the past, dyskinetic areas and dilation were predominant, and volume reduction was relatively easy to perform. More recently, akinesia became the most diffuse morphological aspect. Akinetic areas are present in more than 70% of the patients who undergo SVR. However, these patients present worse hemodynamic parameters with lower LV compliance. Reduction of distensibility increases the end-diastolic pressures (and, consequently, the pulmonary pressures) and affects the remote zones earlier than in patients with dyskinetic areas. When progressive dilation of the uninvolved zone becomes predominant and dilated cardiomyopathy occurs, medical treatment and surgical options, except for heart transplantation, become ineffective and temporary. The extent of the dilation is often not uniform. The involvement of the septum and anterior free wall is often different because of the anatomy of the branches of the left anterior descending coronary artery. Diagonal branches originate often at 45°; as a consequence, the involvement of the anterior free wall is triangular, with the apex in the upper portion. Septal branches originate often at 70–90°; as a consequence, the involvement of the septum starts as high as the anterior free wall but is deeper than it. The septum then bulges toward the right ventricle, minimizing the external dilation. This anatomic aspect has become more common. This technique is to address the correction mainly to the septum, which is rebuilt in such a way to be moved anteriorly; the longitudinal axis is maintained as long as possible to maintain a conical shape. However, when the scar is limited to the apical portion of the septum and the anterior wall, a classic Dor procedure with or without a patch will guarantee the maintenance of the conical shape because it is applied to the distal part of the LV. Conventional goals during reconstruction of the left ventricle in patients with ischemic heart disease and anteroseptal scars were directed toward excluding scars. However, retention of the spherical shape might persist when patch placement is limited to the scar rim, resulting in a smaller cavity and a more spherical heart. LV sphericity can further progress in the months after surgical intervention. Fluid dynamics in more spherical ventricles are impaired, and reduction of both volume and wall stress alone can be insufficient to improve function.

Pocar also showed that the Dor procedure left a less elliptical chamber than reported when "shape or form" became the surgical goal [39]. To achieve a more conical chamber after anterior infarction, elliptical shape reconstruction guidelines must create an apex and narrow the mid-wall by placing either direct sutures or a patch beyond the scar-related end point, form rather than disease is selected as the surgical goal. A fundamental conceptual change follows this observation, as sutures to form an ellipse must be placed to create the apex and normal or non-scarred muscle within the high septum just below the aortic valve. Addressing normal muscle rather than only disease fosters natural opposition, but evolution must be linked to data instead of the reaction. When addressing only the scar, the wider mid-walls are maintained which define a higher ESVI or raised equatorial dimension markers. By contrast, the creation of a conical chamber by employing a patch or using only direct sutures would construct an elliptical form by developing a "curtain" within LV to rebuild a more cone-shaped LV chamber; this approach simply rearranges the apex and mid-wall elements to achieve a more normal sphericity index of 0.5.

This concept of restoring the physiological ventricular ellipse has been further refined by Parachuri et al. [2, 3]. One hundred and two consecutive patients with post-transmural myocardial infarctions were subjected to linear endoventricular patch plasty (EVLPP).

Surgical Technique of EVLPP

We modified the technique of endoventricular patch plasty, by making the patch linear to address the dyskinetic/akinetic area, and adding a Teflon-buttressed linear repair to the ventriculotomy site. The LV cavity was opened by a linear incision parallel to the LAD. The residual LV cavity was assessed visually. We did not use any residual LV cavity measuring devices, as we believe that the accuracy of measurement by these devices is fallacious in the cardiopleged heart. A 3 × 10 cm linear hemashield patch was used for LV reconstruction. Demarcation of the infarct zone was not done. A linear patch was sutured to the border zone into the LV cavity which excluded the infracted areas of the myocardium with an oblique lie from base to apex (Fig. 6.15). This patch was not preformed and hence was individualized to each ventricular volume and geometry. With the rectangular patch sutured to the border zone, the uninfarcted myofibers forming the anterior and anterolateral ventricular walls were reoriented to an oblique orientation from their horizontal position. The aneurysmal apex was excluded by creating a neo-apex with a smaller radius of curvature. The ventriculotomy site was closed with a Teflon-buttressed linear repair. Concomitant CABG was performed in 19 (35.7%) patients using 1 ± 1.2 grafts and mitral valve repair with an annuloplasty ring in 8 (15%) patients for grade 2+ mitral regurgitation.

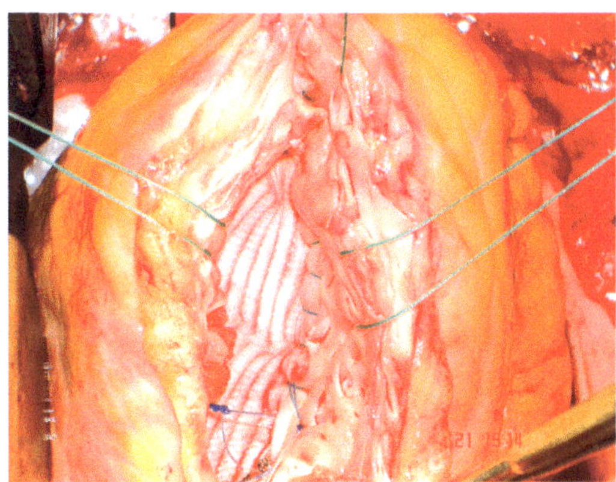

Fig. 6.15 The linear endoventricular patch which excludes the scarred myocardium (With permission from Parachuri et al. [2]. Copyright Elsevier)

We found a 31% decrease in ESVI following surgery with an additional decrease of 5.4% in ESVI at 2 years, signifying persistent reverse remodeling with absence of re-remodeling. The sphericity index also showed significant improvements following surgery and demonstrated further significant improvements at 2 years (Table 6.1). The patient characteristics and results have been detailed in further chapters.

As is evident, medical therapy alone for left ventricular aneurysm has so far proven unpersuasive with a significantly large mortality and morbidity affecting quality of life. Hence, surgical restoration of the adversely remodeled ventricle is necessary for improving quality of life. The area of asynergy contains significant amounts of scar or fibrotic tissue, despite areas of viable

Table 6.1 LV geometry (echocardiography)

Preoperative	Post-op (30 days)	2-year follow-up	*p* value
LVEF: 31.5%±6.5%	34.2%±5.9%	38.4%±4.5%	$p<0.001$
LVIDd: 60.2±7.5 mm	55±7 mm	51.2±6.6 mm	$p<0.001$
LVIDs: 48.1±7.9 mm	43.4±7.7 mm	38.4±6.9 mm	$p<0.001$
EDV: 140.3±38.3 mL	100.8±3.5 mL	68.4±12.4 mL	$p<0.001$
ESV: 95.1±26.1 mL	66±21.7 mL	54.2±16.4 mL	$p<0.001$

myocardium scattered within it. Revascularization alone does not improve clinical outcomes as reported by a randomized multicenter trial [46], the details of which will be discussed in the ensuing chapters.

The techniques of surgical ventricular restoration have undergone a steady evolution from the 1950s to now, wherein the emphasis shifts from mere volume reduction to optimal restoration of physiological ventricular shape. The surgical techniques discussed here portray the limitations of conventional wisdom in dealing with this subset of very sick patients. Hence, rethinking is required into the fundamental concept of function following form which has been oft emphasized by various scientists and clinicians.

References

1. Glower DD, Lowe JE. Left ventricular aneurysm. In: Cohn LH, Edmunds Jr LH, editors. Cardiac surgery in the adult. New York: McGraw-Hill; 2003. p. 771–88.
2. Parachuri VR, Adhyapak SM, Kumar P, Setty R, Rathod R, Shetty DP. Ventricular restoration by linear endoventricular patchplasty and linear repair. Asian Cardiovasc Thorac Ann. 2008;16:401–6.
3. Adhyapak SM, Parachuri VR. Lessons from a mathematical hypothesis: modification of the endoventricular circular patch plasty. Eur J Cardiothorac Surg. 2011;39:945–51.
4. Favoloro RG, Effler DB, Groves LK, Westcott RN, Suarez E, Lozada J. Ventricular aneurysm – clinical experience. Ann Thorac Surg. 1968;6:227–45.
5. Likhoff W, Bailey CP. Ventriculoplasty: excision of myocardial aneurysm. J Am Med Assoc. 1955;158: 915.
6. Walker WE, Stoney WS, Alford Jr WC, Burus GR, Frist RA, Glassford DM. Techniques and results of ventricular aneurysmectomy with emphasis on anteroseptal repair. J Thorac Cardiovasc Surg. 1978;76:824–31.
7. Jatene AD. Left ventricular aneurysmectomy. J Thorac Cardiovasc Surg. 1985;89:321–31.
8. Dor V, Saab M, Coste P, et al. Left ventricular aneurysm: a new surgical approach. Thorac Cardiovasc Surg. 1989;37:11–9.
9. Cox JL. Surgical management of left ventricular aneurysms by the Jatene technique. Oper Techn Cardiothor Surg. 1997;2:117–24.
10. Jatene AD. Surgical treatment of left ventricular aneurysm. In: Baue AE, Geha AS, Hammond GL, Laks H, Naunheim KS, editors. Glenn's thoracic and cardiovascular surgery, vol. 2. 5th ed. Norwalk: Appleton & Lange; 1991. p. 1829–36.
11. Dor V. Surgical management of left ventricular aneurysms by the endoventricular circular patch plasty technique. Oper Techn Cardiothor Surg. 1997;2:139–50.
12. Dor V, Sabatier M, Di Donato M, et al. Late hemodynamic results after left ventricular patch repair associated with coronary grafting in patients with post-infarction akinetic or dyskinetic aneurysm of the left ventricle. J Thorac Cardiovasc Surg. 1995;110: 1291–301.
13. Menicanti L, Di Donato M. The Dor procedure: what has changed after fifteen years of practice? J Thorac Cardiovasc Surg. 2002;124:886–90.
14. Mickleborough LL, Maruyama H, Liu P, et al. Results of left ventricular aneurysmectomy with a tailored scar excision and primary closure technique. J Thorac Cardiovasc Surg. 1991;107:690–8.
15. Mickleborough LL. Left ventricular aneurysm: modified linear closure technique. Oper Techn Cardiothor Surg. 1997;2:118–31.
16. Lundblad R, Abdelnoor M, Svennevig JL. Surgery for left ventricular aneurysm: early and late survival after simple linear repair and endoventricular patch plasty. J Thorac Cardiovasc Surg. 2004;128:449–56.
17. Shapira Oz M, Davidoff R, Hilkert RJ, Aldea GS, Fitzgerald CA, Shemin RJ. Repair of left ventricular aneurysm: long-term results of linear repair versus endoaneurysmorrhaphy. Ann Thorac Surg. 1997;63: 701–5.
18. Parolari A, Naliato M, Loardi C, Denti P, Trezzi M, Zanobini M, Porqueddu M, Roberto M, Kassem S, Alamanni F, Tremoli E, Biglioli P. Surgery of left ventricular aneurysm: a meta-analysis of early outcomes following different reconstruction techniques. Ann Thorac Surg. 2007;83:2009–16.
19. Klein P, Bax JJ, Shaw LJ, Feringa HH, Versteegh MI, Dion RA, Klautz RJ. Early and late outcome of left ventricular reconstruction surgery in ischemic heart disease. Eur J Cardiothorac Surg. 2008;34: 1149–57.

20. Faxon DP, Myers WO, McGabe CH, Davis KB, Schaff HV, Wilson JW, Ryan TJ. The influence of surgery on the natural history of angiographically documented left ventricular aneurysm: the Coronary Artery Study. Circulation. 1986;74(Suppl):I110–8.
21. Di Mattia DG, Di Biasi P, Salati M, Mangini A, Fundarò P, Santoli C. Surgical treatment of left ventricular post-infarction aneurysm with endoventriculoplasty: late clinical and functional results. Eur J Cardiothorac Surg. 1999;15:413–8.
22. Dor V, Sabatier M, Di Donato M, Maioli M, Toso A, Montiglio F. Late hemodynamic results after left ventricular patch repair associated with coronary grafting in patients with postinfarction akinetic or dyskinetic aneurysm of the left ventricle. J Thorac Cardiovasc Surg. 1995;110:1291–301.
23. Dor V, Sabatier M, Di Donato M, Montiglio F, Toso A, Maioli M. Efficacy of endoventricular patch plasty in large postinfarction akinetic scar and severe left ventricular dysfunction: comparison with a series of large dyskinetic scar. J Thorac Cardiovasc Surg. 1998;116:50–9.
24. Dor V, Saab M, Coste P, Kornazewska M, Montiglio F. Left ventricular aneurysm: new surgical approach. J Thorac Cardiovasc Surg. 1989;37:11–9.
25. Fundaro P, Pocar M, Marchetto G, Moneta A, Mattioli R, Donatelli F, Grossi A. Early surgical anteroseptal ventricular endocardial restoration after acute myocardial infarction. Pathophysiology and surgical considerations. Ital Heart J. 2003;4:252–6.
26. Menicanti L, Di Donato M, Frigiola A, Buckberg G, Santambrogio C, Ranucci M, Santo D, RESTORE Group. Ischemic mitral regurgitation: intraventricular papillary muscle imbrication without mitral ring during left ventricular restoration. J Thorac Cardiovasc Surg. 2002;123:1041–50.
27. Mills NL, Everson CT, Hockmuth DR. Technical advances in the treatment of left ventricular aneurysm. Ann Thorac Surg. 1993;55:792–800.
28. Ueno T, Sakata R, Igura Y, Yamamoto H, Ueno M, Ueno T, Matsumoto K. Mid-term changes of left ventricular geometry and function after Dor, SAVE, and overlapping procedures. Eur J Cardiothorac Surg. 2007;32:52–7.
29. Raman J, Dixit A, Bolotin G, Jeevanandam V. Failure modes of left ventricular reconstruction or the Dor procedure: a multiple-institutional perspective. Eur J Cardiothorac Surg. 2006;30:347–52.
30. Cirillo M, Amaduci A, Quaini E, Villa E, Tomba MD, Mhagna Z, Brunelli F, Messina A, Troise G. Patch size, shape and orientation affect geometrical outcomes of surgical anterior ventricular restoration. J Cardiovasc Med (Hagerstown). 2008;9:389–95.
31. Di Donato M, Sabatier M, Menicanti L, Dor V. Incidence of ventricular arrhythmias after left ventricular reconstructive surgery. J Thorac Cardiovasc Surg. 2007;133:289–91.
32. Buckberg GD. Congestive heart failure: treat the disease, not the symptom – return to normalcy. J Thorac Cardiovasc Surg. 2001;121:628–37.
33. Mickleborough LL, Carson S, Ivanov J. Repair of dyskinetic or akinetic left ventricular aneurysm: results obtained with a modified linear closure. J Thorac Cardiovasc Surg. 2001;121:675–82.
34. Buckberg GD. Questions and answers about the STICH trial: a different perspective. J Thorac Cardiovasc Surg. 2005;130:245–9.
35. Menicanti L, Di Donato M, Castelvecchio S, Santambrogio C, Montericcio V, Frigiola A, Buckberg G, RESTORE group. Functional ischemic mitral regurgitation in anterior ventricular remodeling: results of surgical ventricular restoration with and without mitral repair. Heart Fail Rev. 2004;9: 317–27.
36. Enriquez-Sarano M, Schaff HV, Frye RL. Mitral regurgitation: what causes the leakage is fundamental to the outcome of valve repair. Circulation. 2003;108: 253–6.
37. Grigioni F, Enriquez-Sarano M, Zehr KJ, Bailey KR, Tajik AJ. Ischemic mitral regurgitation: long term outcome and prognostic implications with quantitative Doppler assessment. Circulation. 2001;103: 1759–64.
38. Vural KM, Sener E, Ozatik MA, Taşdemir O, Bayazit K. Left ventricular aneurysm repair: an assessment of surgical treatment modalities. Eur J Cardiothorac Surg. 1998;13:49–56.
39. Pocar M, Di Mauro A, Passolunghi D, Moneta A, Alsheraei AM, Bregasi A, Mattioli R, Donatelli F. Predictors of adverse events after surgical ventricular restoration for advanced ischaemic cardiomyopathy. Eur J Cardiothorac Surg. 2010;37: 1093–100.
40. Di Donato M, Dabic P, Castelvecchio S, Santambrogio C, Brankovic E, Collarini L, Joussef T, Frigiola A, Buckberg GD, Menicanti L, RESTORE group. Left ventricular geometry in normal and post-anterior myocardial infarction patients: sphericity index and 'new' conicity index comparisons. Eur J Cardiothorac Surg. 2006;29:225–30.
41. Buckberg GD, Weisfeldt ML, Ballester M, Beyar R, Burkhoff D, Coghlan HC, Doyle M, Epstein ND, Gharib M, Ideker RE, Ingels NB, LeWinter MM, McCulloch AD, Pohost GM, Reinlib LJ, Sahn DJ, Sopko G, Spinale FG, Spotnitz HM, Torrent-Guasp F, Shapiro EP. Left ventricular form and function scientific priorities and strategic planning for development of new views of disease. Circulation. 2004;110: 333–6.
42. Calafiore AM, Iacò AL, Amata D, Castello C, Varone E, Falconieri F, Bivona A, Gallina S, Di Mauro M. Left ventricular surgical restoration for anteroseptal scars: volume versus shape. J Thorac Cardiovasc Surg. 2010;139:1123–30.
43. Suma H, Isomura T, Horii T, Nomura F. Septal anterior ventricular exclusion procedure for idiopathic dilated cardiomyopathy. Ann Thorac Surg. 2006;82: 1344–8.
44. Cooley DA. Repair of the calcified ventricular aneurysm. Ann Thorac Surg. 1990;49:489–90.

45. Guilmet D, Popoff G, Dubois C, Tawil N, Bachet J, Goudot B, et al. Nouvelle technique chirurgicale pour la cure des aneurysmes du ventricule gauche: l'aneurysmoplastie en paletot. Resultats preliminaires. 11 observations. Arch Mal Coeur Vaiss. 1984;77: 953–8.
46. Jones RH, Velazquez EJ, Michler RE, STICH hypothesis 2 investigators. Coronary bypass surgery with or without surgical ventricular restoration. N Engl J Med. 2009;360(17):1705–17.
47. Mickleborough LL, Merchant N, Provost Y, Carson S, Ivanov J. Ventricular reconstruction for ischemic cardiomyopathy. Ann Thorac Surg. 2003;75:S6–12.
48. Reddy SB, Cooley DA, Duncan JM, Norman JC. Left ventricular aneurysm: twenty-year surgical experience with 1572 patients at the Texas Heart Institute. Cardiovasc Dis. 1981;8(2):165–86.
49. Calafiore AM, Di Mauro M, Di Giammarco G, Gallina S, Iacò AL, Contini M, Bivona A, Volpe S. Septal reshaping for exclusion of anteroseptal dyskinetic or akinetic areas. Ann Thorac Surg. 2004;77:2115–21.

The Surgical Technique of Linear Endoventricular Patch Plasty

7

V Rao Parachuri, Chiran Babu, Vineet Mahajan, and Srilakshmi M. Adhyapak

Introduction

The concept of surgically restoring the ventricle to a near-normal physiologic geometry has been the goal of successful treatment of advanced heart failure due to left ventricular aneurysms following transmural myocardial infarctions [1]. The resulting geometry after surgical restoration has concerned a number of surgeons since the first successful repair in 1958, but little attention was placed on the altered geometry until attempts were made to effect a more physiologic aneurysmorrhaphy in 1973. Substantial attention was focused on a concept of geometric reconstruction from within the left ventricle in 1985 [2]. A prosthetic patch was employed with the concept to redirect normal muscle bundles to their original orientation and position. Further refinements include use of improved materials for the repair, preservation, and bypass of the left anterior descending coronary artery, ablation of ventricular arrhythmias when indicated, and the absence of prosthetic material used in contact with the pericardial surface. The previous chapters have dealt with the innovations in surgical technique which has led to an evolution toward greater normalcy in the restored ventricular geometry.

Here, we discuss our technique of linear endoventricular patch plasty (EVLPP) which restores the left ventricular geometry to near normal [3, 4].

Principles of EVLPP

- To restore left ventricular geometry to a normal physiological geometry by restoring its elliptical form.
- Incise the akinetic or aneurismal dyskinetic area from apex to base depending on the extent of the transmural scar irrespective of scar location.
- Unlike other techniques of surgical ventricular restoration (SVR), the left ventricular geometry is restored to a more elliptical one by EVLPP by excluding the infarct from apex to base inclusive of the septum and free wall of the LV.
- The length and width of the endoventricular patch are dictated by the extent of myocardial scar.
- We do not use ventricular cavity measuring devices as they can be fallacious in the cardiopleged heart. We instead rely on visual

V R. Parachuri, FRCS (CTh) (✉)
Heart Lung Transplantation Program,
Narayana Hrudayalaya Institute of Medical Sciences,
258/A, Bommasandra Industrial Area, Anekal Taluk,
Bangalore, Karnataka 560099, India
e-mail: hellorao@gmail.com

C. Babu, A MCh • V. Mahajan, MCh
Department of Cardiothoracic Surgery,
Narayana Hrudayalaya Institute of Medical Sciences,
258/A, Bommasandra Industrial Area, Anekal Taluk,
Bangalore 560099, Karnataka, India
e-mail: chiran_babu@hotmail.com;
vmcardtho@yahoo.com

S.M. Adhyapak, DNB
Department of Cardiology,
St. John's Medical College Hospital,
Sarjapura Road, Bangalore, Karnataka 560034, India
e-mail: srili2881967@yahoo.com

V R. Parachuri, S.M. Adhyapak, *Ventricular Geometry in Post-Myocardial Infarction Aneurysms*,
DOI 10.1007/978-1-4471-2861-8_7, © Springer-Verlag London 2012

estimation of the scar extent. We also do not plicate the transitional zone by any means. The widespread use of the Fontan suture for plication of the transitional zone decreases the ventricular volume but increases ventricular sphericity. It creates a smaller but more spherical ventricle. The use of a linear endoventricular patch ensures an ellipsoid restoration of the ventricle.

- Finally, linear repair with Teflon strips is added to the edges of the ventriculotomy to stabilize the underlying repair and for ensuring hemostasis.

Between 2001 and 2006, EVLPP was performed in 102 patients aged 25–75 years, with a mean age of 43.2 ± 8.3 years. There were 82 men and 20 women, of whom 60% were in New York Heart Association (NYHA) functional class IV.

Inclusion criteria were previous transmural myocardial infarction (MI), significant LV dilatation with LV end-systolic volume index ≥60 mL·m^{-2} with large akinetic or dyskinetic segments. Most patients (95%) presented with cardiac failure, of whom 28% also had angina, and 5% presented with ventricular tachyarrhythmias. There was no incidence of thromboembolism. The location of the aneurysm was anterior due to anterior myocardial infarction (MI) in 95 patients and inferior in 7 with inferior MI. There were 65 patients with diabetes.

The left ventricular volumes were assessed by 2D transthoracic echocardiography and transesophageal echocardiography. The residual left ventricular volume was also assessed by the preoperative transesophageal echocardiography and preoperative contrast ventriculography. Although MRI and 3D echocardiography are more sensitive and specific for left ventricular volume assessment in the presence of large aneurysms which are akinetic or dyskinetic [5], we could not use MRI and 3D echocardiography due to logistic constraints. However, in patients where the left ventricular endocardial borders were not clearly defined by 2D transthoracic echocardiography, we used contrast echocardiography for more specific delineation of the LV endocardial borders to facilitate accurate left ventricular volume measurements. This method has been validated as being as accurate as MRI assessment for LV volumes [6].

Surgical Procedure

Repair of Anterior Left Ventricular Aneurysms

Under general anesthesia, after endotracheal intubation, the patient is prepared and draped (see Video 7.1). Routine monitoring lines are introduced: right radial arterial line, right internal jugular vein central venous line, and Swan Ganz catheter to monitor pulmonary artery pressures.

A transesophageal echocardiography probe is inserted after intubation to delineate left ventricular clots, mitral valve morphology, and function of the remote myocardium. The contractility of remote myocardium is assessed by 2D echocardiography and centerline analysis of contrast ventriculography in the right anterior oblique view before surgery.

After median sternotomy, the pericardium is opened vertically and marsupialized. The ascending aorta is cannulated with appropriate arterial and two-stage single venous cannula. In case of additional mitral valve repair or repair of inferior aneurysms, bicaval cannulation is accomplished. The aorta is cross clamped and both antegrade and retrograde cold blood cardioplegias are administered to maintain moderate hypothermia at 28°C.

The myocardial surface is examined for extent of scar with simultaneous visual assessment of remote myocardium (Fig. 7.1). An incision is made vertically 2–3 cm to the left of the left anterior descending coronary artery (Fig. 7.2a, b). This incision starts just above the cardiac apex and extends toward the cardiac base. The extent of the incision is dictated by the extent of the scar which is palpated between the surgeon's right index finger positioned within the left ventricular cavity and the surgeon's right thumb placed on the anterior surface of the LV.

Generally, the superior extent of the incision is limited by the free muscle bundle arising

Video 7.1 Repair of anterior left ventricular aneurysm by linear endoventricular patch plasty

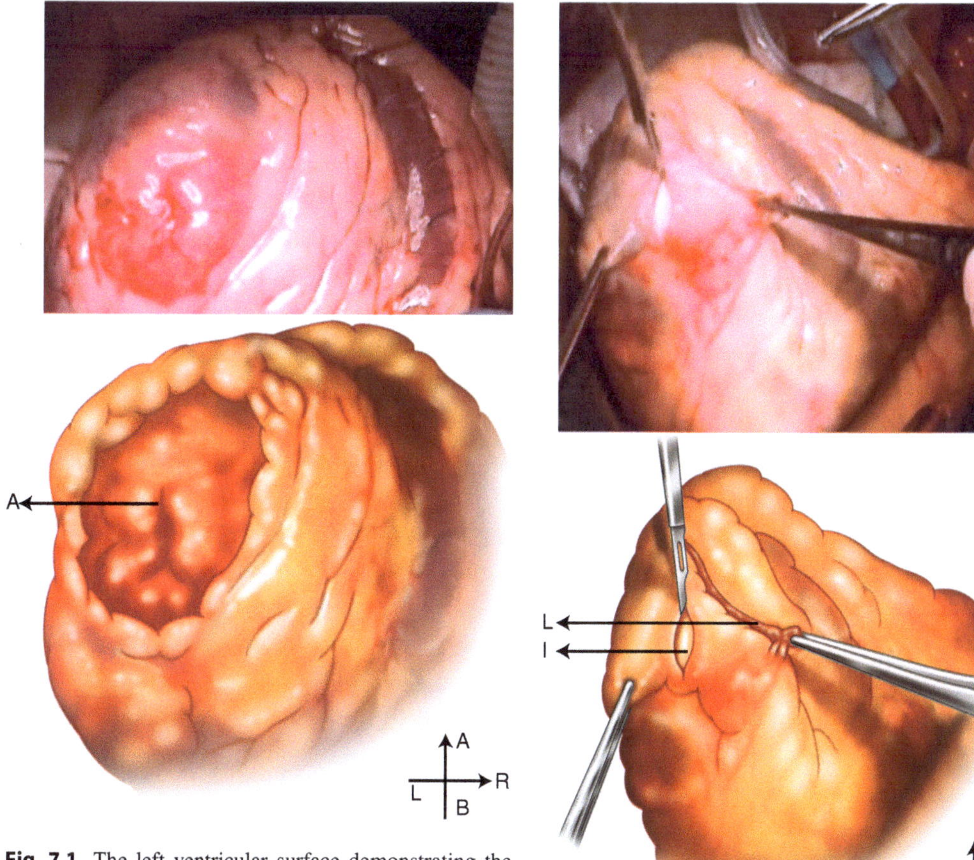

Fig. 7.1 The left ventricular surface demonstrating the scarred area. *A* apex

Fig. 7.2 The left ventriculotomy incision parallel to the left anterior descending coronary artery. *I* incision, *L* left anterior descending coronary artery

from the anterior LV free wall adjacent to the anterolateral papillary muscle and inserting into the interventricular septum (Fig. 7.3a, b). This muscle bundle may have to be divided in order to further extend the ventriculotomy toward the ventricular base. This muscle bundle is a feature in nearly all patients.

Next, four stay sutures are deployed at the apex, base, lateral edge of the LV opening, and medial edge of the LV opening to expose the LV cavity adequately (Fig. 7.4a, b). The LV cavity is now examined thoroughly. Assessment is made of anomalous muscle bundles, LV clots, position of papillary muscles, and extent of infarct into the septum and apex. The small apical interlacing muscles are divided and clots are removed. Thorough suction is applied to the LV cavity, left atrium, around the mitral leaflets, and proximal aorta in order to remove any small thrombi which have gravitated during initial handling of the heart. If cryoablation is indicated, it is performed at this stage (details in Chap. 11) (Fig. 7.23).

A woven Dacron graft of size 30 mm or more, out of which a rectangular patch is made (of about 6- to 8-cm length and 2- to 4-cm width) (Fig. 7.5a, b). This is used as the endoventricular patch, and in accordance to the extent of the scar is not performed. Instead, it gets modelled into the LV cavity depending on the extent of infarct. The width is therefore chosen in such a way as to approximate the uninfarcted septum to the healthy anterior wall by incorporating the endoventricular patch without compromise to the residual LV cavity.

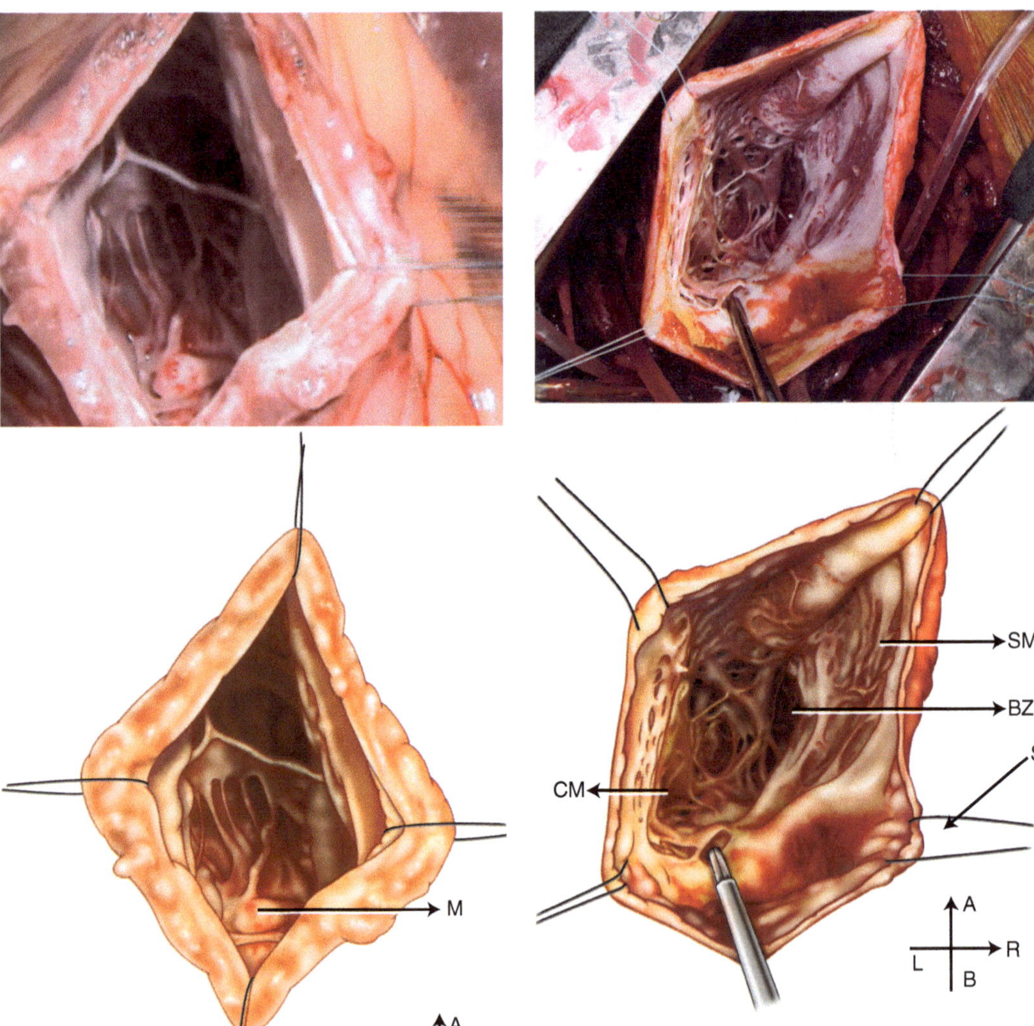

Fig. 7.3 The LV cavity visualized through the ventriculotomy demonstrating the free muscle bundle and myocardial scar. *M* muscle bundle from lateral LV wall toward apex

Fig. 7.4 The LV cavity opened through the ventriculotomy. *CM* contractile muscle, *SM* scarred muscle, *BZ* border zone, *S* suture

The patch is sutured from the ventricular base with pledgetted 3-0 polypropylene sutures positioned medial to the anterolateral papillary muscle in its lateral extent and sutured toward the apex (Fig. 7.6). Care should be taken not to include the base of the anterolateral papillary muscle. On the medial extent of the patch, it is sutured to the transition zone at the border between the infarcted muscle and uninfarcted myocardium in the septum. If the septal involvement is more extensive, with a large septal scar, the sutures in the septum are placed more anteriorly to avoid compromising the residual LV cavity.

At this stage, the inferior extent of the patch is measured up to the lower end of the ventriculotomy incision and is cut (Fig. 7.7a, b). This region corresponds to the neoapex. A second suture is used to exclude the infarcted ventricular apex. The lower end of the patch is sutured to this end. On the left side, a running suture excludes the infarcted zone and joins the first suture. Here, care is taken to avoid the base of the posteromedial

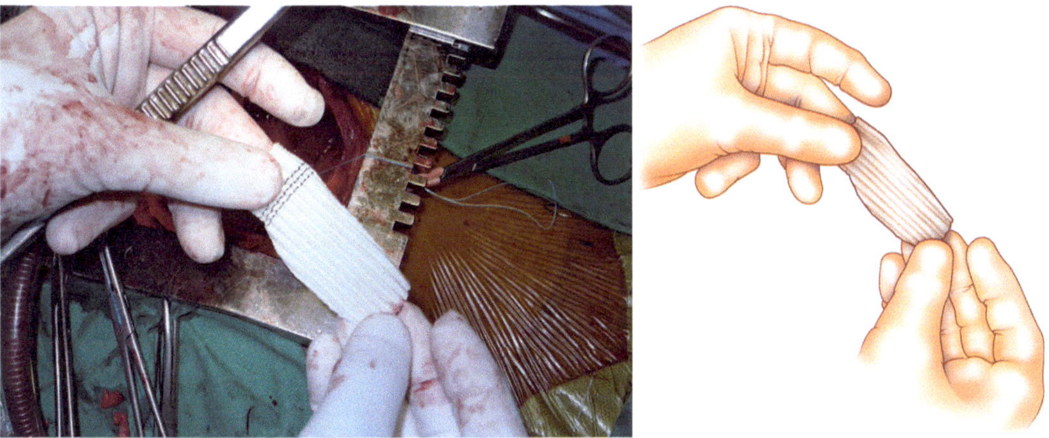

Fig. 7.5 The linear endoventricular woven Dacron patch

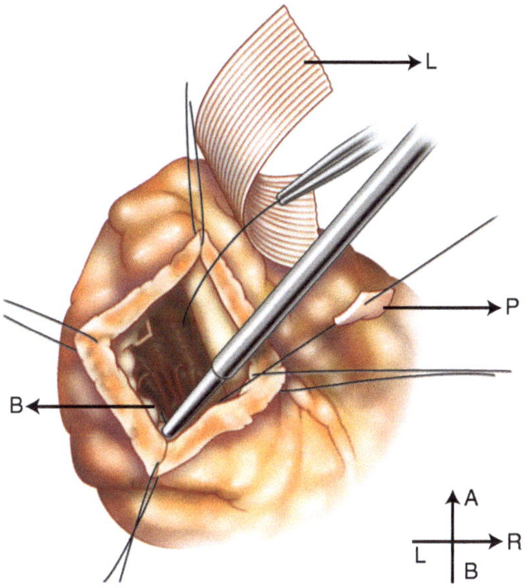

Fig. 7.6 Pledgetted suture *P* used to anchor the linear patch *L* to the endocardium at the base of the heart *B*.

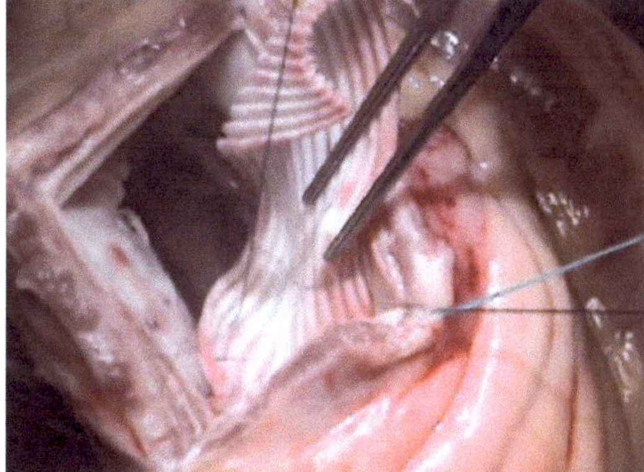

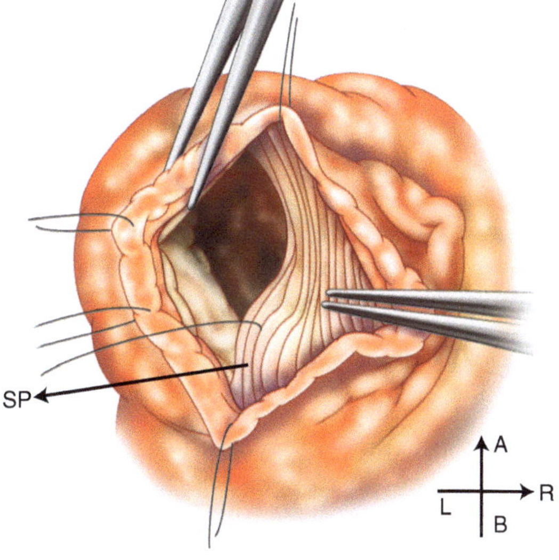

Fig. 7.7 Suturing of linear endoventricular patch to the LV free wall

papillary muscle. The other end of the suture runs on the septal surface excluding the infarcted cardiac apex, running at the transition zone toward the first suture with which it is tied (Figs. 7.8, 7.9 a, b 7.10a, b 7.11, and 7.12).

The residual LV cavity is not measured by any measuring device. A visual assessment is employed, and the maintenance of an adequate residual LV cavity is accomplished by keeping the endoventricular patch geometry linear, avoiding

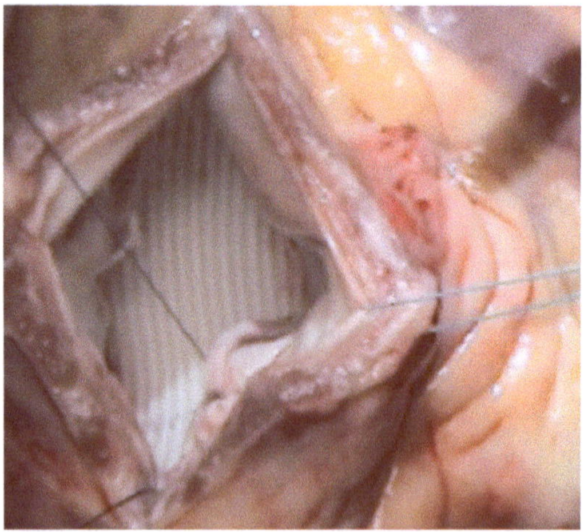

Fig. 7.8 Suturing of the linear endoventricular patch to the septal side of the LV

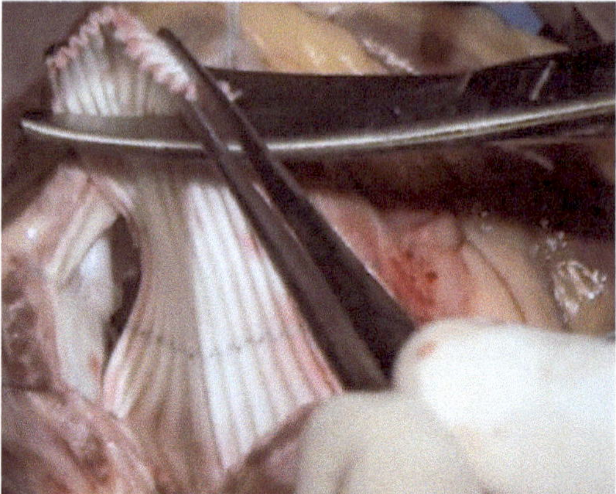

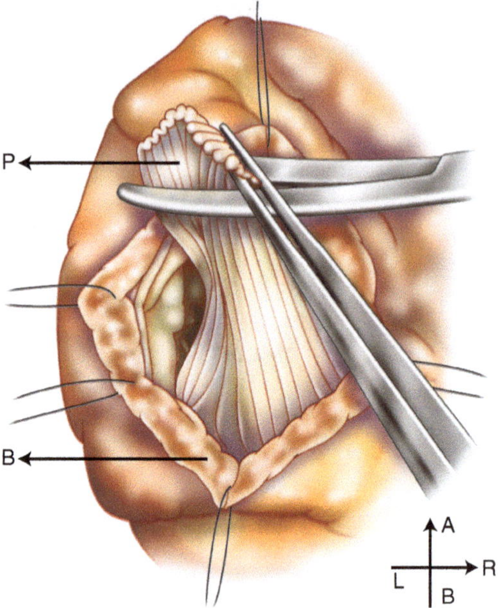

Fig. 7.9 Tailoring of the graft length keeping the apical end of the incision as a reference. *P* linear endoventricular patch, *B* base of the ventricle

plication of the transition zone and by keeping adequate distance from the bases of the anterolateral and posteromedial papillary muscles and with recruiting just enough scarred septal area.

For larger aneurysms, wider endoventricular patches of up to 4-cm width are used.

After anchoring the endoventricular patch, additional sutures are placed to prevent leaks (Fig. 7.13). Closure of the ventriculotomy is done in a linear fashion buttressed by two hard Teflon felt strips applied on either side of the ventriculotomy edges (Fig. 7.14a, b) and sutured in two layers. A deeper interrupted horizontal mattress suture using 2-0 polypropylene is employed with a superficial over and over incorporating the Teflon strips with 2-0 polypropylene suture (Figs. 7.15, 7.16).

Repair of Inferior Left Ventricular Aneurysms

Inferior wall aneurysms are repaired similarly, but the septal scar involvement is not as extensive as in anterior aneurysms. Unlike in anterior LV aneurysms, the inferior LV aneurysms have scars which have sharply demarcated borders separating them from uninfarcted healthy myocardium. The LV is opened approximately 2 cm lateral to the posterior descending coronary artery. The cavity was visually assessed to locate the posteromedial papillary muscle (generally spared from the aneurysm), and the linear woven Dacron patch is sutured to the rim of noninfarcted tissue between the scarred aneurysm and the myocardium from base to apex. The scar in inferior LV aneurysms tends to involve the LV base more extensively. Hence, care should be taken not to involve the mitral valve apparatus while suturing the linear endoventricular patch at the base. Besides, care needs to be taken not to involve the base of the posteromedial papillary muscle (Fig. 7.17). The length of the patch is

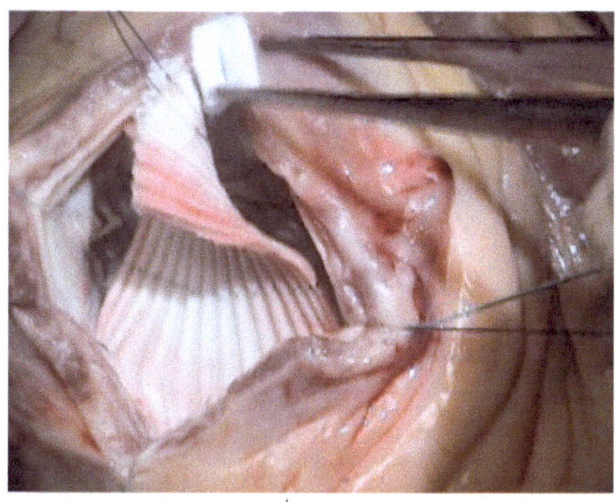

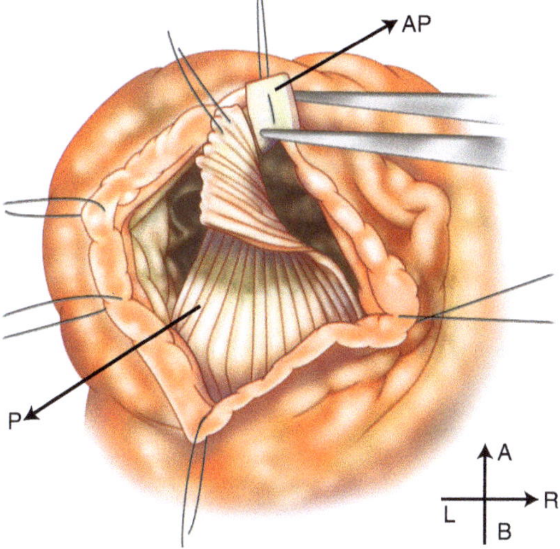

Fig. 7.10 Creation of a neoapex by suturing of the apical end of the endoventricular patch to exclude the scarred *LV* apex. *AP* apical pledget, *P* linear endoventricular patch

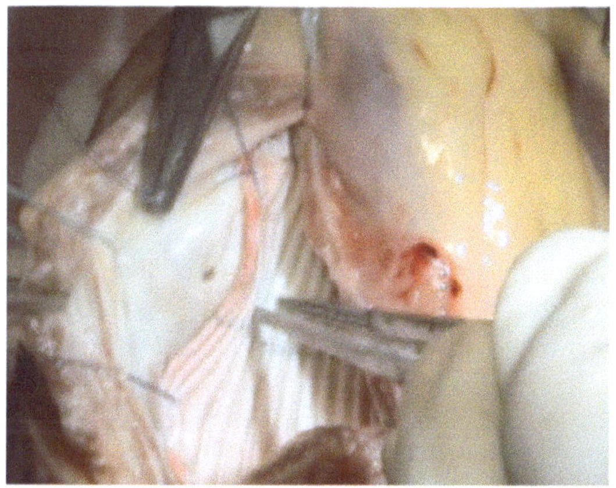

Fig. 7.11 Suturing of the patch from the apex to the free wall

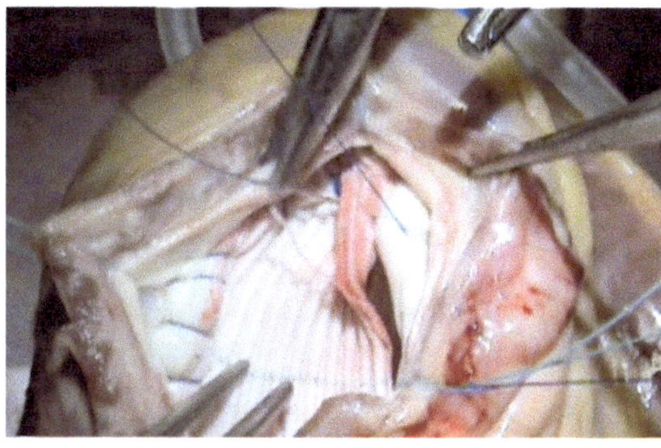

Fig. 7.12 Suturing of the endoventricular patch from the apical end towards the ventricular base at the septal side

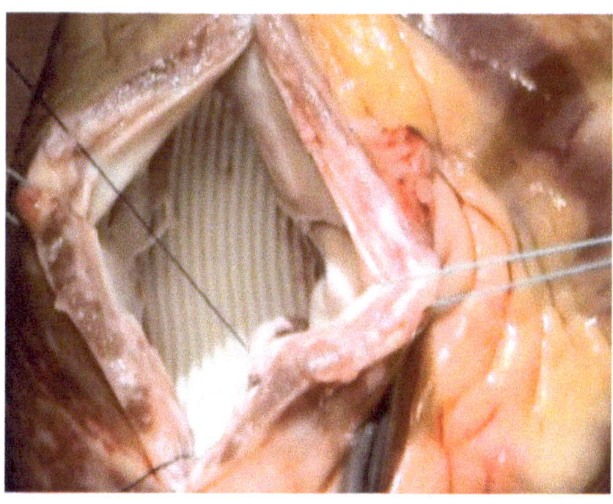

Fig. 7.13 Completed linear endoventricular patch plasty. Position of the sutured linear endoventricular patch which excludes the infarcted muscle from noninfarcted muscle

adjusted to the length of the scar toward the apex and excessive patch is trimmed. This is followed by a Teflon-buttressed linear repair at the ventriculotomy site (Fig. 7.18).

Repair of Lateral Left Ventricular Aneurysms

Repair of lateral wall LV aneurysms are also accomplished by similar means. The ventriculotomy incision is from base to apex in the region of the scar tissue. Here, too, the scar tissue is sharply demarcated from surrounding uninfarcted tissue. The linear endoventricular patch

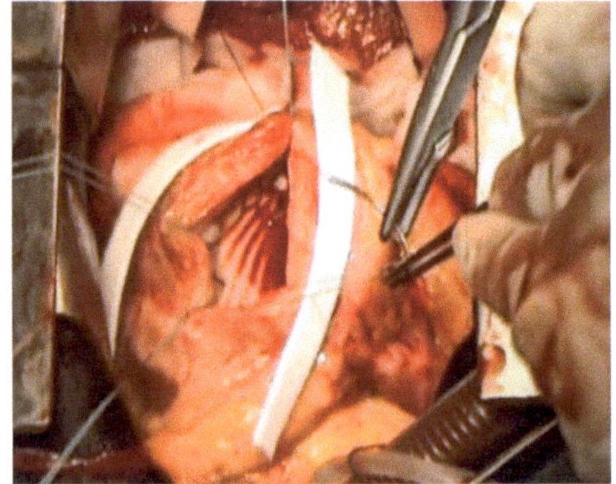

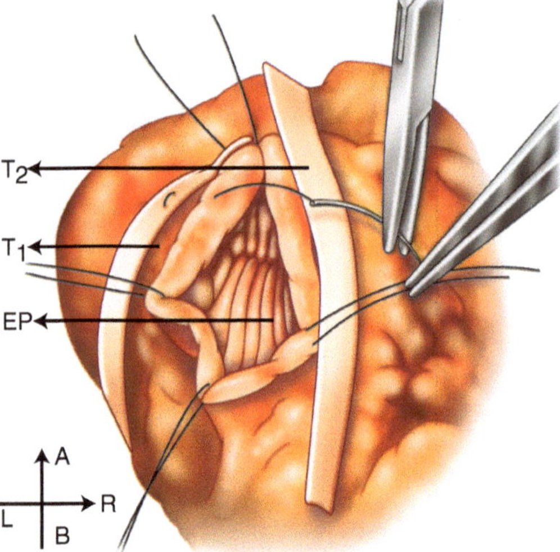

Fig. 7.14 The ventriculotomy being closed buttressed by two Teflon strips on either side and sutured in two layers of mattress sutures (**b**). *EP* endoventricular patch, T_1 Teflon strip on the *left* of the ventriculotomy, T_2 Teflon strip to the *right* of the ventriculotomy

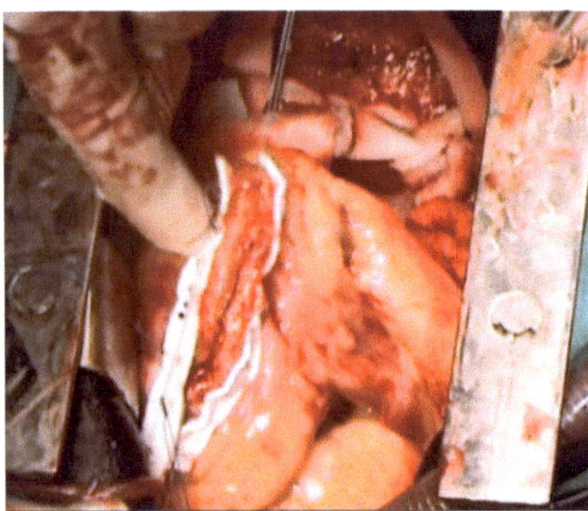

Fig. 7.15 Ventriculotomy closure with horizontal matress sutures

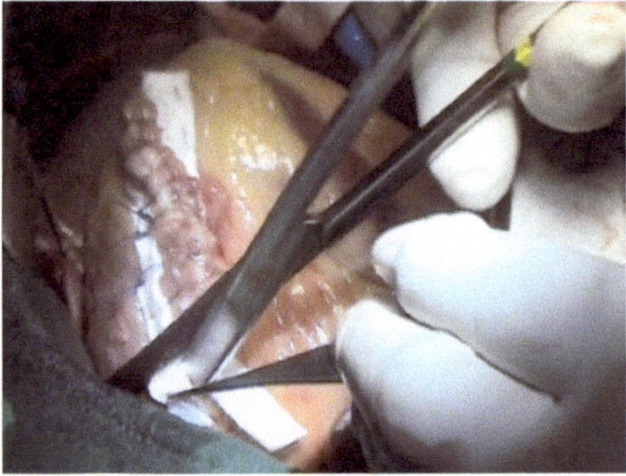

Fig. 7.16 Final ventriculotomy closure with final over and over suture completed with trimming of the excess Teflon strip

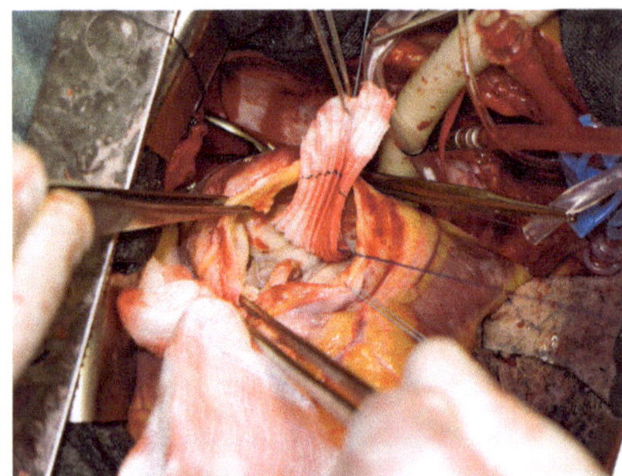

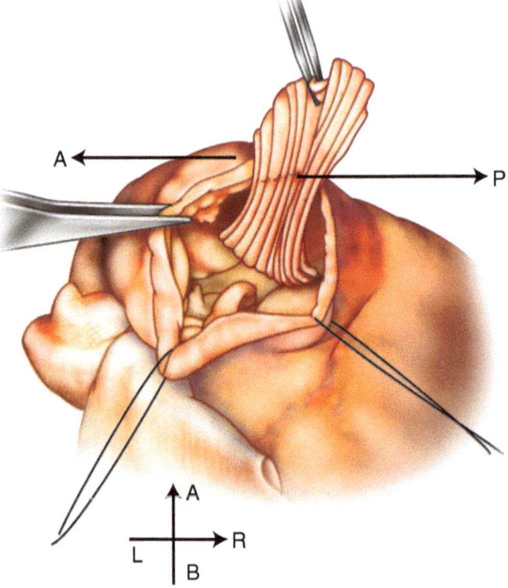

Fig. 7.17 Repair of an inferior *LV* aneurysm. *A* apex, *P* endoventricular patch

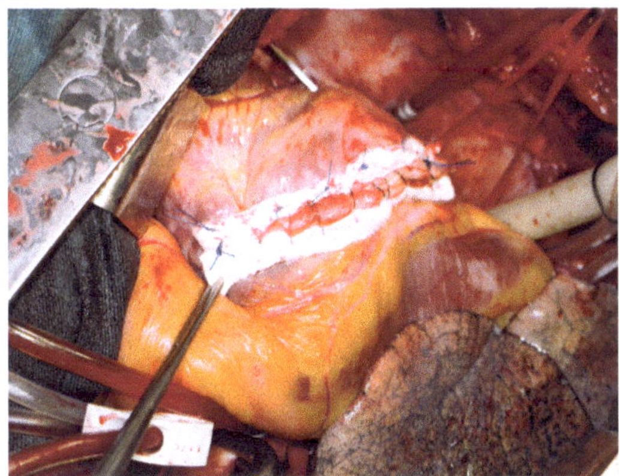

Fig. 7.18 Closure of inferior ventriculotomy after repair of inferior lv aneurysm

is sutured similarly from base to apex, taking care to avoid damage to the base of the posteromedial papillary muscle. Again here, the scar extends into the ventricular base to a greater extent than anterior scars. The excess patch is trimmed toward the ventricular apex. This is followed by a Teflon-buttressed linear repair at the site.

Additional revascularization is always accomplished by use of internal mammary or saphenous venous graft in cases of occluded LAD. Although, the myocardium supplied by the LAD has been excluded, it is important to revascularize the portion supplied by the proximal LAD and its first septal branch. This area sometimes is not involved by scar and therefore constitutes viable but ischemic myocardium.

Mitral valve repair is accomplished through the left atrium with a rigid Carpentier Edwards mitral annuloplasty ring (details in Chap. 12). This technique of EVLPP maintains an ellipsoid geometry of the left ventricle and also realigns the papillary muscles which have been displaced farther by scar tissue and ventricular dilatation. Our patients with absent preoperative mitral regurgitation did not develop mitral regurgitation even late after surgery. The benefits of late reverse remodeling is evident by this technique [3, 4].

After completion, rewarming is started, with de-airing through the aortic root and ventriculotomy. The aortic cross clamp is released followed by incremental increase in preload, and the patient is weaned off cardiopulmonary bypass. The further need for intra-aortic balloon counterpulsation and inotropes is judged by hemodynamic assessment and instituted accordingly.

Repair of Postinfarction Ventricular Septal Rupture

A certain group of patients with postinfarction ventricular septal rupture who present late with symptoms and signs of advanced heart failure are primarily repaired by surgical ventricular restoration and ventricular septal rupture closure at our institution. We have not repaired acute postinfarction VSRs by surgical ventricular restoration and concomitant VSR closure. The few survivors of postinfarction ventricular septal rupture presenting at 4–6 weeks following the acute myocardial infarction, with advanced congestive heart failure and dyskinetic areas in the apex and distal septum and distal anterior wall, are chosen for repair. The idea of this technique of repair is to prevent the occurrence of congestive heart failure due to large areas of dyskinesia. We had two patients with postinfarction VSR who presented at 1 and 10 years after postinfarction VSR closure with advanced heart failure due to dyskinesia of apex, distal septum, and distal anterior wall. The VSR patch in them was intact. These patients underwent successful surgical ventricular restoration by the technique described above at our institution. These patients prompted us to primarily repair postinfarction VSR presenting late, that is after 6 weeks by surgical ventricular restoration and concomitant VSR closure.

The left ventriculotomy is accomplished under cardiopulmonary bypass, 2–3 cm lateral to the LAD, in anterior infarcts. The ventricle is inspected for the defect/defects, amount, and extent of infarcted muscle and intramural thrombi. After debriding the thrombus, the defect is closed with a glutaraldehyde-fixed autologous pericardial patch using continuous 3-0 polypropylene sutures (Fig. 7.19). Next, the infarct is excluded from the uninfarcted myocardium using a 4×10-cm linear rectangular woven Dacron patch which is sutured from the ventricular base,

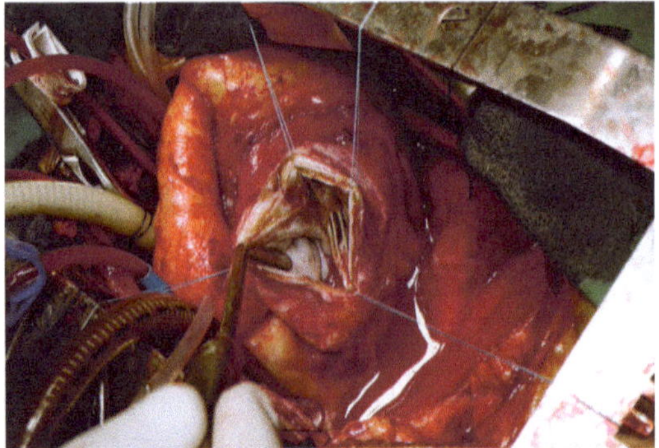

Fig. 7.19 Repair of inferior aneurysm with vsr. the sucker is placed through the vsr

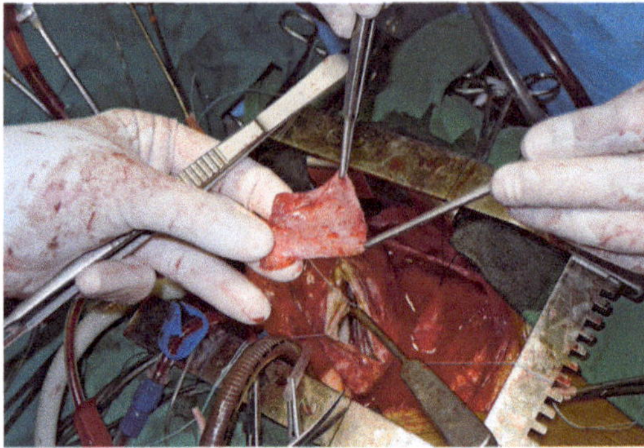

Fig. 7.20 The ventricular septal defect is closed by the pericardial patch. *P* pericardial patch, *A* ventricular apex

staying medial to the lateral papillary muscle base and extending toward the apex, using continuous 3-0 polypropylene sutures (Figs. 7.20, 7.21, and 7.22). The medial border of the Dacron patch is usually below the pericardial patch closure of the ventricular septal rupture. This accomplishes near total exclusion of the infarct with complete repair of the ventricular septal defect, preventing even tiny residual shunts. Sometimes the LAD may not be graftable due to friability, mid-LAD lesions, or small caliber of the vessel. The ventriculotomy site is then closed with Teflon strips using interrupted pledgetted sutures in a linear fashion.

In patients with posterior septal defects and inferior aneurysms, the repair is accomplished similarly with closure of the defects using glutaraldehyde-fixed autologous pericardial patch and a linear woven Dacron patch for exclusion of the inferior areas of dyskinesia. Care is taken while suturing the Dacron patch at the mitral annulus and the posteromedial papillary muscle. The rest of the procedure is accomplished as described previously. Our procedure of arrhythmia surgery for patients presenting with ventricular tachycardia was linear cryoablation which is described in detail in Chap. 11 using the surgical cryoprobes described (Figs. 7.23).

Our clinical results and hemodynamic results have been detailed in Chap. 8.

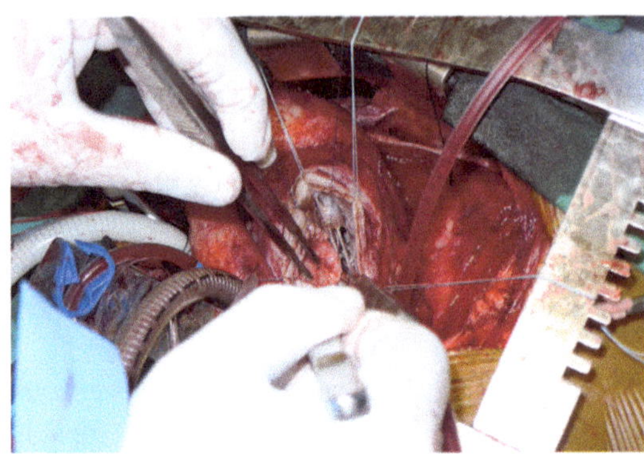

Fig. 7.21 Vsr closed with pericardial patch. After closure of the ventricular septal defect with autologous pericardium, the LV aneurysm is being excluded by a Dacron linear endoventricular patch

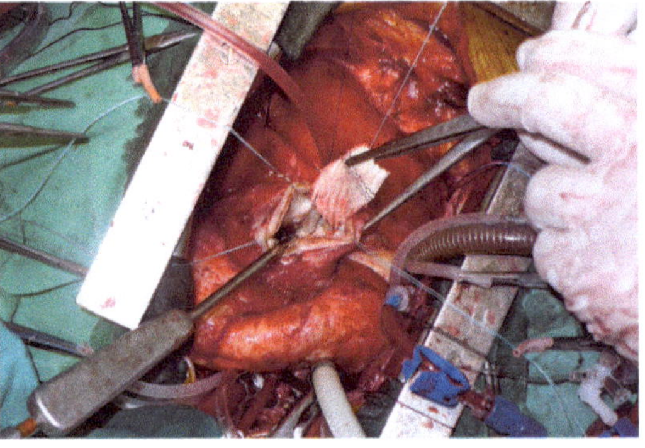

Fig. 7.22 Linear Dacron endoventricular patch used to exclude the aneurysmal area along with the VSD which has been closed by pericardium

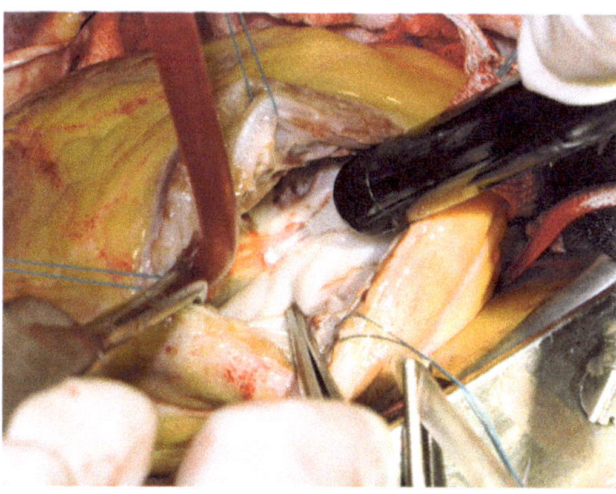

Fig. 7.23 Cryoablation being performed starting at the mitral annulus toward the endoventricular patch on the *left* side in the posterolateral wall of the *left* ventricle in a patient with concomitant ventricular tachycardia

References

1. Likhoff W, Bailey CP. Ventriculoplasty: excision of myocardial aneurysm. J Am Med Assoc. 1955;158:915.
2. Dor V, Saab M, Coste P, et al. Left ventricular aneurysm: a new surgical approach. Thorac Cardiovasc Surg. 1989;37:11–9.
3. Parachuri VR, Adhyapak SM, Kumar P, Setty R, Rathod R, Shetty DP. Ventricular restoration by linear endoventricular patchplasty and linear repair. Asian Cardiovasc Thorac Ann. 2008;16:401–6.
4. Adhyapak SM, Parachuri VR. Lessons from a mathematical hypothesis: modification of the endoventricular circular patch plasty. Eur J Cardiothorac Surg. 2011;39:945–51.
5. Qin JX, Jones M, Shiota T, Greenberg NL, Tsujino H, Firstenberg MS, Gupta PC, Zetts AD, Xu Y, Sun P, Cardon LA, Odabashian JA, Flamm RD, White JA, Panza JA, Thomas JD. Validation of real-time three-dimensional echocardiography for quantifying left ventricular volumes in the presence of a left ventricular aneurysm: in vitro and in vivo studies. J Am Coll Cardiol. 2000;36:900–7.
6. Malm S, Frigstad S, Sagberg E, Larsson H, Skjaerpe T. Accurate and reproducible measurement of left ventricular volume and ejection fraction by contrast echocardiography: a comparison with magnetic resonance imaging. J Am Coll Cardiol. 2004;44:1030–5.

Surgical Ventricular Restoration by the Technique of Endoventricular Linear Patch Plasty: Long-Term Clinical Results

8

Introduction

The role of surgical ventricular restoration (SVR) has been clearly established as an option for treatment of advanced heart failure due to ischemic cardiomyopathy with large aneurysms. Its role is limited in patients with diffusely dilated akinetic ventricles (dilated cardiomyopathy), although Suma et al. [1] have surgically restored large akinetic ventricles using long ellipsoid intraventricular patches. The technique of SVR has been successful only in those patients with large areas of akinesis or dyskinesis, that is, areas of dyssynergy which measure >20% of the ventricular surface area. The existence of viable contractile myocardium is an absolute must for the success of SVR.

The technique of geometric repair betters the technique of classical linear repair [2, 3]. The use of intraventricular patches to exclude the aneurismal area not only restores better ventricular geometry but also allows for performing concomitant procedures like revascularization and mitral valve repair. The long-term results of the endoventricular circular patch plasty (EVCPP) showed evidence of re-remodeling an increase in the end-diastolic volume by 15% from the post-operative values. Besides, MRI studies distinctly showed the restored ventricular geometry to be more spherical than true ellipsoid [4]. The EVCPP was further modified by various cardiac surgeons. Calafiore has proved better clinical results in terms of beneficial ventricular remodeling and resultant improvements in morbidity and mortality with the use of long ellipsoid patches to restore dilated ventricles with aneurysms. Several studies have demonstrated that even with EVCPP (endoventricular circular patch plasty), the restored ventricle retains a spherical configuration with the apical curvature being lesser than normal. This adversely affects cardiac systole and diastole, as the apex does not form an optimal fulcrum for ventricular torsion. Long-term ventricular redilatation or re-remodeling also occurs with EVCPP as mentioned. Parachuri et al. have modified the intraventricular patch geometry to a linear configuration which is not preformed and is sutured to exclude the scarred myocardium. This technique has a mathematical basis and is based on Vayo' mathematical hypothesis of the left ventricular aneurysm. Here, the technique of endoventricular linear patch plasty (EVLPP) and its results are presented.

Mathematical Basis for the Technique of EVLPP

A mathematical model was proposed by Vayo [5] to study the hemodynamics of a left ventricular aneurysm. The ventricle was arbitrarily designated a spherical shape, and the aneurismal area was designated two different shapes: (1) spherical and (2) rectangular (Fig. 8.1). The aneurismal areas were inactive or noncontractile and were subtended by the diameter of their sides forming angles at the center of the sphere. In systole, when the ventricle contracted, the aneurysm remained

V R. Parachuri, S.M. Adhyapak, *Ventricular Geometry in Post-Myocardial Infarction Aneurysms*,
DOI 10.1007/978-1-4471-2861-8_8, © Springer-Verlag London 2012

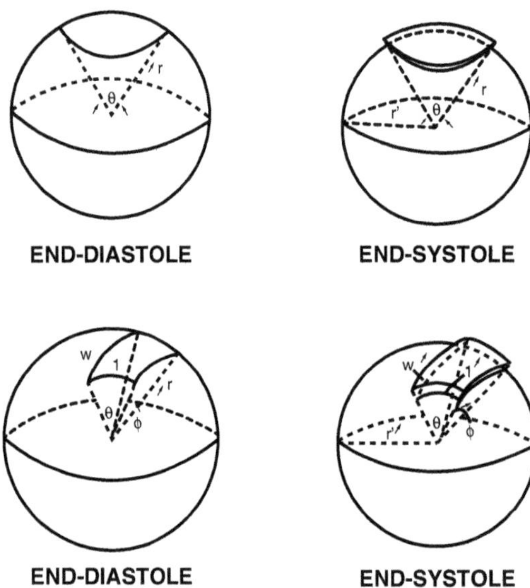

Fig. 8.1 Comparison of circular and rectangular aneurysms in diastole and systole (With permission from Klein et al. [6]. Copyright LWW journals)

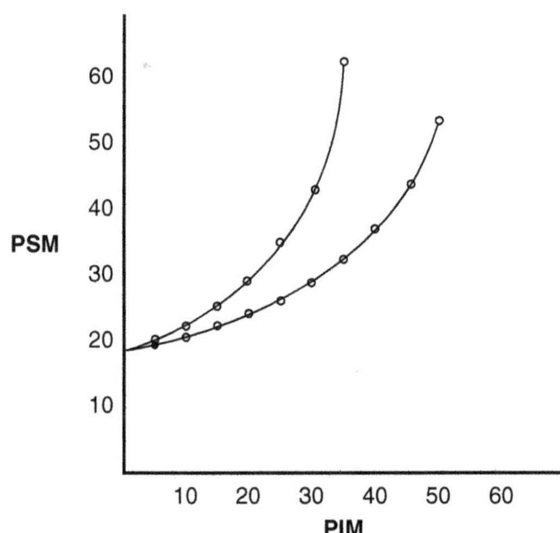

Fig. 8.2 Relationship of percent inactive muscle to percent active muscle between circular and rectangular aneurysms (With permission from Klein et al. [6]. Copyright LWW journals)

noncontractile. There were two assumptions made: (1) contraction of the ventricle was concentric, maintaining constancy of the angles subtending the aneurysm and (2) constant stroke volume.

When the percent contractile muscle was compared with percent inactive muscle, there was a greater ratio of contractile to noncontractile muscle for all sizes of rectangular aneurysms than for circular aneurysms (Fig. 8.2).

But when the aneurismal area was 30% of the ventricular surface area, the values could not be computed, as the stroke volume fell precipitously low. This is because, as the noncontractile area reaches 25% of total ventricular surface area, the ventricle has to dilate in order to maintain an effective forward stroke volume.

Based on this mathematical hypothesis, the endoventricular patch was modified to a 3 × 10-cm linear/rectangular geometry and was sutured to the border zone within the ventricular cavity excluding the infarcted myocardium as far as possible. The demarcation of the border zone by the Fontan suture was abandoned, as this increased the sphericity of the restored ventricle. The use of measuring devices for residual ventricular cavity measurement was also avoided, as this could be fallacious in the cardiopleged heart. Thus, the ventricle was surgically restored by using a linear/rectangular endoventricular patch of <25% of the ventricular surface area.

Patients and Methods

Between 2001 and 2006, SVR was performed in 102 patients aged 25–75 years, with a mean age of 43.2 ± 8.3 years. There were 82 men and 20 women, of whom 60% were in New York Heart Association (NYHA) functional class IV. *Inclusion criteria* were previous transmural myocardial infarction (MI), significant LV dilatation with LV end-systolic volume index ≥60 mL·m^{-2} with large akinetic, or dyskinetic segments. Most patients (95%) presented with cardiac failure, of whom 28% also had angina; 5% presented with ventricular tachyarrhythmias. There was no incidence of thromboembolism. The location of the aneurysm was anterior due to anterior myocardial infarction (MI) in 95 patients and inferior in 7 with inferior MI. There were 65 patients with diabetes.

The left ventricular volumes were assessed by 2D transthoracic echocardiography and transesophageal echocardiography. The residual left ventricular volume was also assessed by the

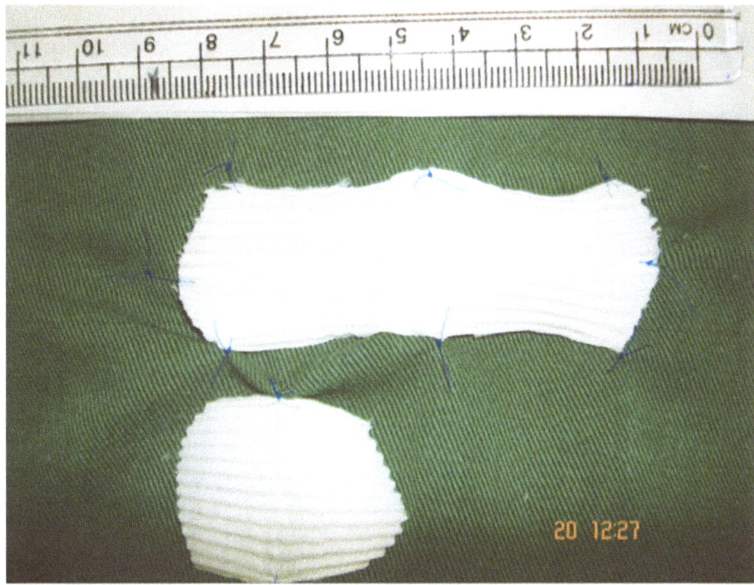

Fig. 8.3 Comparison of the circular and linear endoventricular patches (With permission from Parachuri et al. [9])

preoperative transesophageal echocardiography and preoperative contrast ventriculography. Although MRI and 3D echocardiography are more sensitive and specific for left ventricular volume assessment in the presence of large aneurysms which are akinetic or dyskinetic [7], we could not use MRI and 3D echocardiography due to logistic constraints. However, in patients where the left ventricular endocardial borders were not clearly defined by 2D transthoracic echocardiography, we used contrast echocardiography for more specific delineation of the LV endocardial borders to facilitate accurate left ventricular volume measurements. This method has been validated as being as accurate as MRI assessment for LV volumes [8].

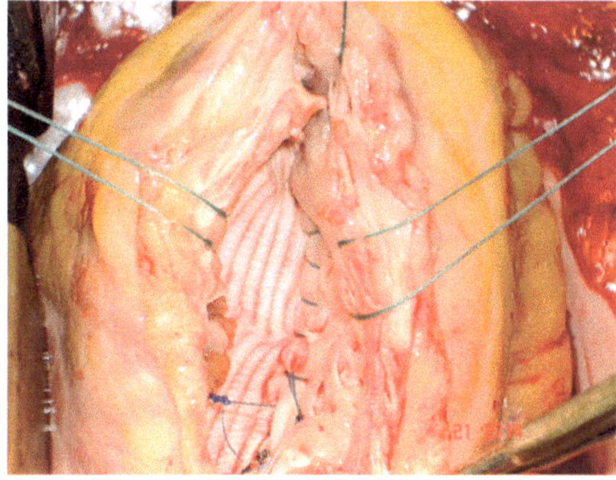

Fig. 8.4 Linear endoventricular patch sutured within the ventricular cavity (With permission from Parachuri et al. [9])

Surgical Technique

A linear 8–12-cm LV incision was made parallel to the left anterior descending coronary artery, 2–3 cm lateral to it, from the base to the apex of the heart. No LV cavity measuring devices were used as we consider them inaccurate during cardioplegia; we relied instead on visual assessment of the residual LV cavity. For the same reason, we do not advocate plication of the border zone by Fontan suture, as this increases the sphericity of the ventricle. We used a linear patch described below (Fig. 8.3). A 3×10-cm linear Hemashield patch was sutured inside the LV cavity, starting from the base toward the apex, using 3/0 Prolene (Fig. 8.4). The length of the patch was tailored to the extent of the infarct from base to apex, usually 6–10 cm. The patch was placed laterally anterior to the anterior papillary muscle. On the medial side, as much as possible of the infarcted septum was excluded without compromising the residual LV cavity. The patch lay obliquely, being molded to the LV cavity. Toward the apex, a neoapex was

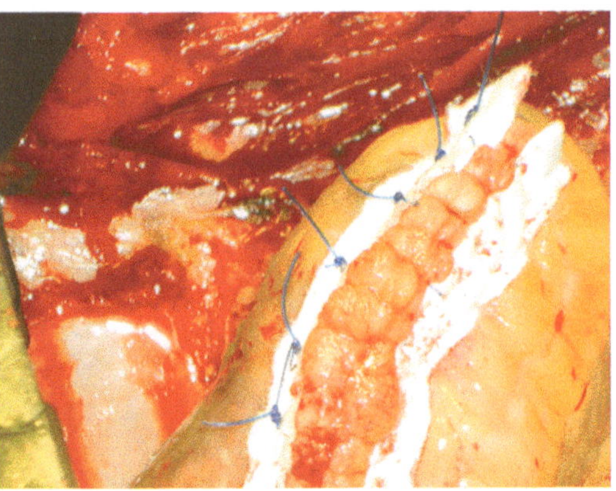

Fig. 8.5 The linear repair over the linear endoventricular patch repair (With permission from Parachuri et al. [9])

created by excluding the aneurysmal apex. The ventriculotomy was closed using a linear repair in two layers, buttressed with Teflon strips (Fig. 8.5). Inferior wall aneurysms were repaired similarly, but the scar did not involve the septum. The LV was opened approximately 2 cm lateral to the posterior descending artery. The cavity was visually assessed to locate the posteromedial papillary muscle (generally spared from the aneurysm), and a linear Hemashield patch was sutured to the rim of noninfarcted tissue between the scarred aneurysm and the myocardium. This was followed by a Teflon-buttressed linear repair at the ventriculotomy site. Concomitant procedures included coronary artery bypass grafting in 73 (77.6%) patients, mitral valve repair for significant (≥Grade II) regurgitation in 39 (41.4%), using Alfieri repair in 19, and a rigid annuloplasty ring in 20. Post-MI ventricular septal defect repair was also performed in three patients, and cryoablation for ventricular tachycardia or fibrillation in six.

Centerline Analysis on Contrast Ventriculography

Here, motion is measured along 100 chords drawn perpendicular to a line constructed midway between the end-diastolic and end-systolic contours on the left ventriculogram in 30° right anterior oblique projection. The measured motion of the 100 chords is normalized for heart size by dividing it by the length of the end-diastolic perimeter. As normal motion varies from chord to chord, the normalized motion at each chord is converted into units of normal standard deviations from the normal mean motion at each chord. Wall motion in each of five regions of the LV contour is determined by averaging the motion abnormality (expressed as standard deviation) of chords 1–16, 17–32, 33–48, 49–64, and 65–80, corresponding to the anterobasal, anterolateral, apical, inferior, and posterobasal regions, respectively. The hypokinetic chords are designated a negative value and hyperkinetic chords are designated a positive value [10].

Left Ventricular Shape Analysis

The EDVI and ESVI were measured following surgery from contrast ventriculography in the RAO projection. These volumes were also calculated based on the formula of volume of an ellipse [11]. Normal values of the left ventricle obtained from age-, sex-, and body surface area-matched controls were substituted for diameter (d) at the ventricular base and apex to base length (h) into the formula for the volume of a prolate ellipsoid, namely, $V = \pi/6d^2h$. The ventricular shape analysis was performed which was modeled on the technique used by Kass and coworkers [12]. The digitized LV contour was traced in systole and diastole. The center moment of the digitized contour was calculated, and using this as origin, radii were drawn to each of the digitized points on the perimeter of the contour. The length of each radius (r) and the angle (θ) relative to a given orientation were measured, and an $r(\theta)$ function was generated. The first digitized point (aortic valve-anterobasal wall intersection) was chosen as the 0° position and was continued counterclockwise from that location to generate a polar representation.

Clinical Results and Evidence of Long-Term Reverse Ventricular Remodeling

Hospital mortality after SVR was 7.8% (eight patients). This included a patient with post-MI ventricular septal rupture who had been in low

Table 8.1 Univariate analysis of prognostic factors for early mortality and low cardiac output

Variable	Mortality	Low output
Sex	≥0.05	0.003
Diabetes mellitus	≥0.05	0.04
Congestive heart failure	0.03	0.032
Preoperative NYHA class	0.027	0.04
Absence of angina	0.029	≥0.05
ESVI ≥60 mL·m^{-2}	0.03	0.02
Ejection fraction ≤30%	0.04	≥0.05
Cardiopulmonary bypass >2 h	0.04	≥0.05
Aortic cross clamp time >1 h	0.02	0.01
Coronary artery bypass	≥0.05	0.02
Mitral valve repair	≥0.05	0.03

With permission from Parachuri et al. [9]
ESVI end-systolic volume index, *NYHA* New York Heart Association

cardiac output with multiorgan failure preoperatively. Five patients who underwent concomitant mitral valve repair succumbed in the intensive care unit in the second postoperative week; an intra-aortic balloon pump was required in three of them. The other two patients died from multiorgan failure. Factors analyzed as predictors of early mortality are listed in Table 8.1. Major complications in the early postoperative period included intra-aortic balloon pump use in five patients. It was inserted perioperatively in two due to low cardiac output, based on systolic blood pressure <90 mmHg, low cardiac index, and low urine output. A low cardiac output state developed in 56 (54.9%) patients, of whom 48 were discharged and 8 died. Renal dysfunction occurred in four patients, which was managed conservatively. There were no significant postoperative arrhythmias, and the incidence of postoperative infection was low (11%). Assessment of factors associated with postoperative low cardiac output state is summarized in Table 8.1. Ejection faction in 94 patients increased significantly from 31.5% ± 6.5% before SVR to 34.2% ± 5.9% before discharge from hospital. Left ventricular dimensions and volumes decreased significantly after SVR: left ventricular internal dimension in diastole from 60.2 ± 7.5 to 55 ± 7 mm, LV internal dimension in systole from 48.1 ± 7.9 to 43.4 ± 7.7 mm ($p < 0.001$), end-diastolic volume index from 140.3 ± 38.3 to 100.8 ± 3.5 mL·m^{-2} ($p < 0.001$), and end-systolic volume index from 95.1 ± 26.1 to 66 ± 21.7 mL·m^{-2} ($p < 0.001$). The sphericity index at discharge was 0.79 ± 0.04 ($p < 0.05$). No patient had an excessive reduction in LV volume resulting in diastolic dysfunction, assessed by Doppler echocardiography [9].

We followed up 72 patients over a period of 0–52 months; the other 22 were from outside the country and follow-up was not possible. Mean duration of follow-up was 24 ± 6.1 months. Echocardiography showed further significant reductions in LV dimensions and volumes (all $p < 0.001$): left ventricular internal dimension in diastole from 55 ± 7 to 51.2 ± 6.6 mm, LV internal dimension in systole from 43.4 ± 7.7 to 38.4 ± 6.9 mm, end-diastolic volume index from 100.8 ± 33.5 to 68.4 ± 12.4 mL·m^{-2}, and end-systolic volume index from 66 ± 21.7 to 54.2 ± 16.4 mL·m^{-2}. There was a further improvement in EF from 34.2% ± 5.9% to 38.4% ± 4.5% ($p < 0.001$). Sphericity index improved to 0.62 ± 0.02, which was significantly better than the preoperative value ($p < 0.01$). We assessed 57 patients for LV geometry by contrast ventriculography 6 months after SVR. There was a decrease in hypokinetic segments from 61.1 ± 12.8 to 36.5 ± 14.8 chords and a decrease in akinetic or dyskinetic segments from 32.5 ± 11 to 25 ± 8.1 chords. There were significant improvements in the anterobasal, anterolateral, and posterobasal segments in anterior aneurysms and in posterobasal and inferior segments in inferior aneurysms (Table 8.2), with further decreases in LV volumes and increases in EF from predischarge values, reflecting continuing negative LV remodeling. There were five midterm deaths at 8 ± 1.2 months

Table 8.2 Ventricular performance by angiography in 57 patients

Aneurysm site	Preoperative	Postoperative	*p* value
Anterior aneurysm (*n*=54)			
Anterobasal	−620	−121	<0.01
Anterolateral	−648	−178	<0.001
Apical	−689	−674	≥0.05
Posterobasal	−121	−86	0.03
Inferior	−428	−122	<0.01
Inferior aneurysm (*n*=3)			
Anterobasal	−14	−12	≥0.05
Anterolateral	−22	−18	≥0.05
Apical	−26	−24	≥0.05
Posterobasal	−68	−26	0.04
Inferior	−68	−22	0.01

With permission from Parachuri et al. [9]

Table 8.3 Factors affecting midterm survival

Variable	Survival (%)	*p* value
Female sex (no/yes)	84/82	≥0.05
Diabetes mellitus (no/yes)	92/45	0.01
NYHA class IV (no/yes)	69/37	0.008
Congestive heart failure (no/yes)	89/84	≥0.05
Intra-aortic balloon pump (no/yes)	83/10	0.04
LAD lesion (no/yes)	83/90	≥0.05
ESVI ≥60 mL·m^{-2} (no/yes)	91/43	0.01
Ejection fraction <30% (no/yes)	85/43	0.01
Coronary artery bypass (no/yes)	86/92	≥0.05
Cardiopulmonary bypass >2 h (no/yes)	84/73	0.006
Low cardiac output (no/yes)	88/75	<0.01
Mitral valve repair (no/yes)	85/89	≥0.05

With permission from Parachuri et al. [9]
EVSI end-systolic volume index, *LAD* left anterior descending artery, *NYHA* New York Heart Association

after SVR, confirmed by telephone interview. Two patients suffered sudden cardiac death and three were hospitalized at local hospitals and died of cardiac causes. Results of survival analysis are presented in Table 8.3. The functional capacity in the survivors improved to NYHA class I in 92% and to class II in 8%. Revascularization and mitral valve repair had no effect on early mortality or midterm survival, but they were associated with less frequent low cardiac output. Cardiac failure requiring hospitalization developed in four patients. The interval from SVR to development of cardiac failure was 9.2±1.2 months.

Thus, linear endoventricular patch plasty resulted in a decrease in end-diastolic volume of 40.2 mL (95% confidence interval (CI): 33.6,46.7) and stroke volume of 10.0 mL (95% CI: 6.6,13.5) and increase in ejection fraction of 6.7% (95% CI: 5.5,7.9). There was a further 14% decrease in EDV and SV (30%) at 2 years with increase in EF (20%). There was a persistent significant improvement in sphericity index with no evidence of re-remodeling.

LV Shape Changes Following Linear Endoventricular Patch Plasty

The calculated ESVI obtained by substituting normal ventricular values from age-, sex-, and BSA-matched controls to the formula of the volume of an ellipse was 41 mL (measured ESVI

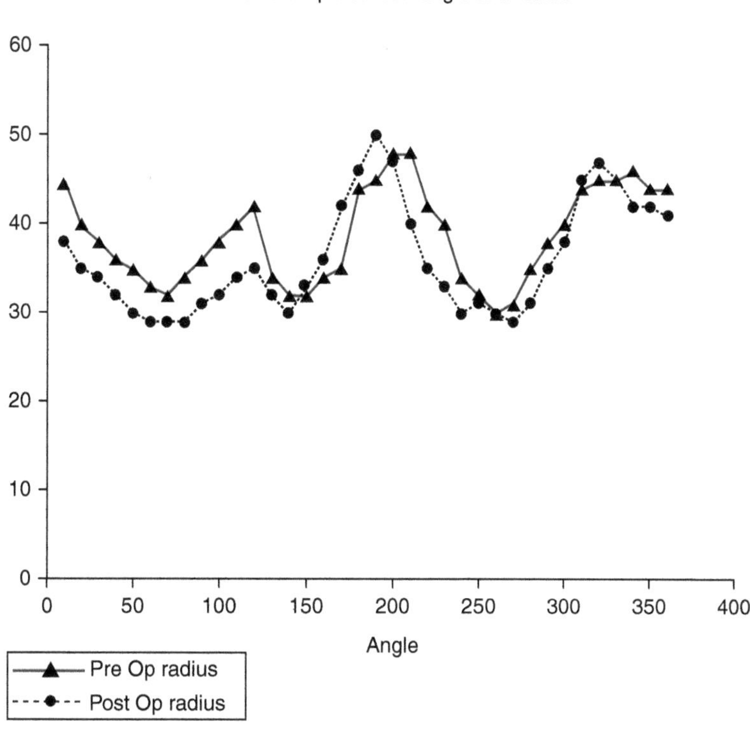

Fig. 8.6 Left ventricular shape analysis of preoperative and postoperative polar representations after linear endoventricular patch plasty (With permission from Adhyapak and Parachuri [13]. Copyright Elsevier)

from postoperative ventriculograms: 48 mL) and the calculated EDVI was 64 mL (measured: 68 mL). Our measured ventricular volumes of the postoperative ventricle thus conform to an ellipsoid geometry. When the preoperative and postoperative polar representations were generated, there were significant decreases in the anterolateral and anterior segments (effect size = 1.1, $p < 0.001$). There was a beneficial change in the inferior segment which did not attain statistical significance ($p = 0.08$). There was no significant change in the inferobasal and anterobasal areas (Fig. 8.6).

The inferobasal and anterobasal areas corresponded to areas of contractile myocardium and hence did not show significant differences following surgery. The apical region also did not show significant differences following surgery. The apex was reconstructed with the linear patch such that a neoapex was formed. As substantial areas of the apex were formed by the akinetic patch, which only moved along with the surrounding myocardium, the shape change in this area was not significant following surgery.

The shape changes following EVCPP have been studied by Fantini and coworkers [14]. They found significant changes in the inferior and inferobasal regions following surgery. The changes in anterior and anterolateral regions were not significant following surgery.

Analysis of the Mancini Curve

The polar representations of the LV contours in systole and diastole when mapped have been named as the "Mancini curve." In the preoperative Mancini curve, the areas subtending the anterolateral and anterior segments of the left ventricle form an angle with the apical region, as these regions are predominantly dyskinetic. The area subtending the apex is rounded and does not have the sharp contour of the normal apex. The areas subtending the inferior and inferobasal regions also form an angle with the apical region as these regions are dyskinetic. This curve represents a predominantly dyskinetic anterior left ventricular aneurysm.

The Mancini curve following EVLPP demonstrates a smoother and more horizontal configuration of the anterolateral and anterior segments of the left ventricle. The apical segment of the curve also demonstrates a more acutely peaked configuration which is similar to the normal Mancini curve although the shape changes in the apical region did not reach statistical significance (Fig. 8.7).

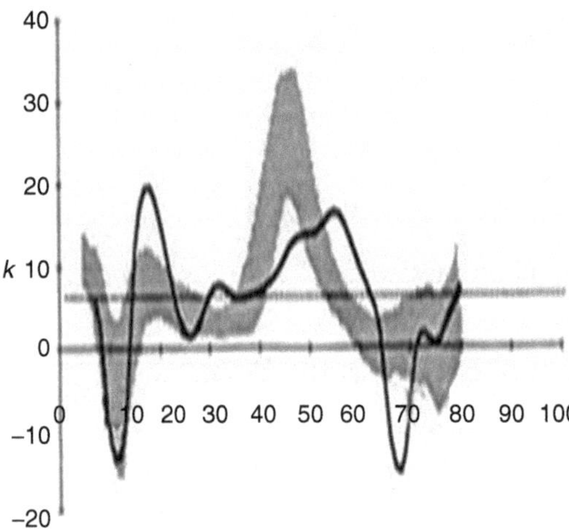

Fig. 8.7 Mancini curve of normal left ventricle (With permission from Mitchell et al. [15])

Relationship of EDVI with the SVI

Following EVCPP, when the percent change in EDVI was compared with percent changes in SVI the relationship was J-shaped (Fig. 8.8). The changes in SVI were not proportional to the EDVI especially for larger decreases in EDVI. This relates to the geometry and size of the non-contractile area in the ventricle, which corresponds to the circular/oval endoventricular patch. When the EDVI is reduced by a large magnitude, with an akinetic circular endoventricular patch, the changes in SVI are not proportional to the changes in EDVI. This also relates to the anatomical substrate of the restored left ventricle, where improvements were only seen in the inferior wall curvature with no change in the anterior wall. The resultant surgically restored ventricle remained spherical albeit with a reduced radius. With EVCPP, the oblique fibers continue to have a slightly horizontal orientation with resultant ineffective systolic shortening reflected by the SVI and contributing to late re-remodeling especially in patients with large pre-operative EDVI.

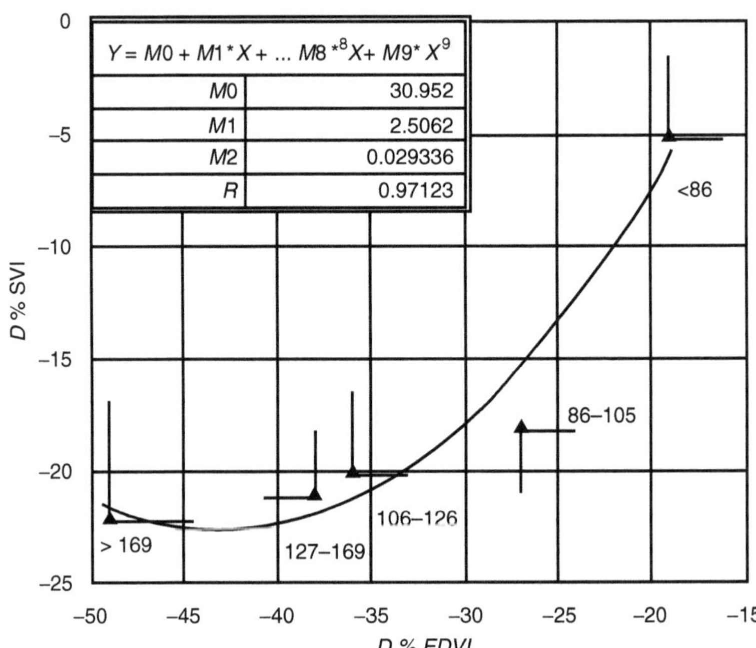

Fig. 8.8 Interaction of percent change in EDVI to percent change in SVI after EVCPP (With permission from Adhyapak and Parachuri [13]. Copyright Elsevier)

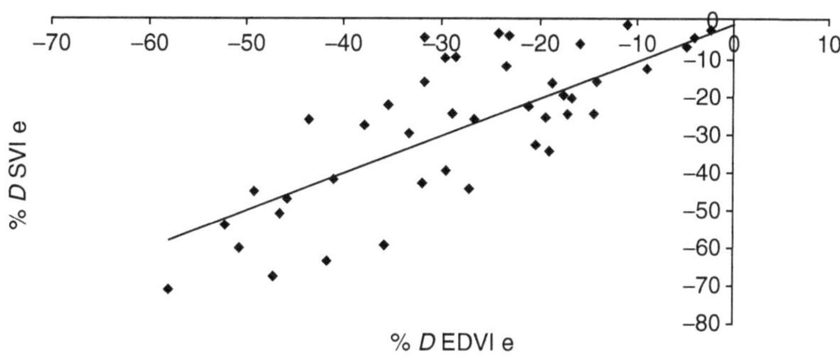

Fig. 8.9 Interaction of percent change in EDVI to percent change in SVI after EVLPP (With permission from Adhyapak and Parachuri [13]. Copyright Elsevier)

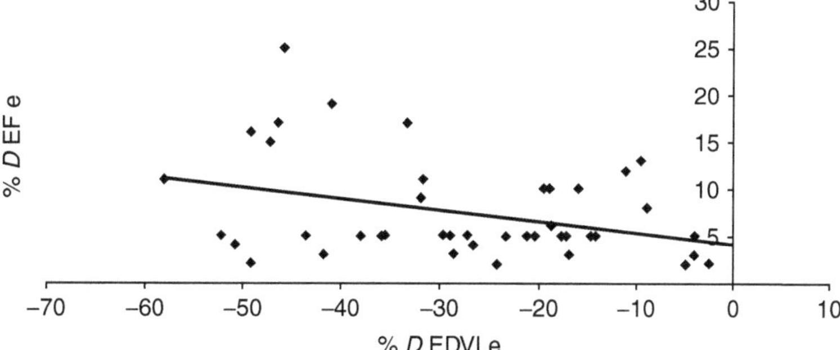

Fig. 8.10 Relationship of percent change in EDVI to percent change in EF after EVLPP (With permission from Adhyapak and Parachuri [13]. Copyright Elsevier)

By modifying the geometry of the endoventricular patch and avoiding the circular Fontan suture used to plicate the neck of the ventricular aneurysm in EVCPP, we found the change in SVI had a significant linear relationship with change in EDVI across all magnitudes of EDVI reduction (Fig. 8.9). This relationship was persistent even 2 years after surgery. Hence, by decreasing the akinetic area to <25% of the ventricular surface area and by configuring its geometry to a linear geometry, the realignment of the anterior and anterolateral ventricular walls is established, resulting in a near-physiological ellipsoid ventricular geometry, while maintaining physiological interactions between the ventricular volumes with persistent late reverse remodeling.

Relationship of EDVI and EF

With EVLPP, there was a significant inverse linear relationship between EDVI and EF across all magnitudes of EDVI decrease early after surgery (Fig. 8.10).

This linearity between EDVI and EF was not present 2 years after EVLPP. The EF has several limitations in assessing LV pump function following SVR. The clinical improvements do not parallel the magnitude of increase in EF. Hence, the linear relationship of the EDVI with SVI which persisted late after EVLPP serves as a marker of physiological ellipsoid LV geometry restoration by this technique.

The Relationship of EDV and SV-Frank Starling Relationship in the Surgically Restored Ventricle

Following SVR, although there was a decrease in SV by 10 mL, there were significant clinical improvements. There was a 31% decrease in ESVI following surgery with an additional decrease of 5.4% in ESVI at 2 years, signifying persistent reverse remodeling with absence of re-remodeling. The occurrence of baseline left ventricular diastolic dysfunction was seen only in those with EDVI >250 mL. Following SVR, the diastolic dysfunction improved from Grade III to Grade I. Despite the paradoxical decrease in stroke volume after SVR with associated improvements in LV geometry and clinical improvements, a significant linear relationship between the EDVI and SVI should be considered a surrogate marker of improvement in LV function after surgery [16, 17].

The surgical technique of EVLPP has clinically validated the mathematical hypothesis of Vayo and by the physiological linearity of relationship of the resting end-diastolic volumes with the stroke volumes at rest.

References

1. Suma H, Isomura T, Horii T, Nomura F. Septal anterior ventricular exclusion procedure for idiopathic dilated cardiomyopathy. Ann Thorac Surg. 2006;82:1344–8.
2. Lundblad R, Abdelnoor M, Svennevig JL. Surgery for left ventricular aneurysm: early and late survival after simple linear repair and endoventricular patch plasty. J Thorac Cardiovasc Surg. 2004;128:449–56.
3. Parolari A, Naliato M, Loardi C, Denti P, Trezzi M, Zanobini M, Porqueddu M, Roberto M, Kassem S, Alamanni F, Tremoli E, Biglioli P. Surgery of left ventricular aneurysm: a meta-analysis of early outcomes following different reconstruction techniques. Ann Thorac Surg. 2007;83:2009–16.
4. Biederman RWW, Doyle M. The contribution of CMR to patients undergoing the surgical ventricular restoration (SVR) procedure; one center's experience over five years. Open Magn Reson. 2009;2:33–45.
5. Vayo HW. Theory of the left ventricular aneurysm. Bull Math Biophys. 1966;28:363.
6. Klein MD, Herman MV, Gorlin R. A hemodynamic study of left ventricular aneurysm. Circulation. 1967;35:614–30.
7. Qin JX, Jones M, Shiota T, Greenberg NL, Tsujino H, Firstenberg MS, Gupta PC, Zetts AD, Xu Y, Sun JP, Cardon LA, Odabashian JA, Flamm SD, White RD, Panza JA, Thomas JD. Validation of real-time three-dimensional echocardiography for quantifying left ventricular volumes in the presence of a left ventricular aneurysm: in vitro and in vivo studies. J Am Coll Cardiol. 2000;36:900–7.
8. Malm S, Frigstad S, Sagberg E, Larsson H, Skjaerpe T. Accurate and reproducible measurement of left ventricular volume and ejection fraction by contrast echocardiography: a comparison with magnetic resonance imaging. J Am Coll Cardiol. 2004;44:1030–5.
9. Parachuri VR, Adhyapak SM, Kumar P, Setty R, Rathod R, Shetty DP. Ventricular restoration by linear endoventricular patch plasty and linear repair. Asian Cardiovasc Thorac Ann. 2008;16:401–6.
10. Sheehan FH, Bolson EL, Dodge HT, Mathey DG, Schofer J, Woo HW. Advantages and applications of the centerline method for characterizing regional ventricular function. Circulation. 1986;74:293–305.
11. Adhyapak SM, Parachuri VR. Architecture of the left ventricle: insights for optimal surgical ventricular restoration. Heart Fail Rev. 2010;15(1):73–83.
12. Kass DA, Traill TA, Keating M, Altieri PI, Maughan WL. Shape changes in aortic and mitral regurgitation: assessment by Fourier shape analysis and global geometric indices. Circ Res. 1988;62(1):127–38.
13. Adhyapak SM, Parachuri VR. Lessons from a mathematical hypothesis: modification of the endoventricular circular patch plasty. Eur J Cardiothorac Surg. 2011;39:945–51.
14. Fantini F, Montiglio F, Sabatier M, Coste P, Barletta G, Donato D. Left ventricular shape changes induced by aneurysmectomy with endoventricular circular patch plasty reconstruction. Eur Heart J. 1994; 15(8):1063–9.
15. Mitchell GF, Lamas GA, Vaughan DE, Pfeffer MA. Left ventricular remodeling in the year after first anterior myocardial infarction: a quantitative analysis of contractile segment lengths and ventricular shape. J Am Coll Cardiol. 1992;19(6):1136–44.
16. Renlund DG, Gerstenblith G, Fleg JL, Becker LC, Lakatta EG. Interaction between end diastolic and end systolic volumes in normal humans. Am J Physiol Heart Circ Physiol. 1990;258(2):H473–81.
17. Adhyapak SM, Parachuri VR. Impact of surgical ventricular restoration on stroke volume: surgical fine tuning of the relationship between end diastolic volume and stroke volume. J Thorac Cardiovasc Surg. 2011;141:1552–3.

The Impact of Surgical Technique on Cardiac Hemodynamics Following Surgical Ventricular Restoration

9

Introduction

The improvements in cardiac anatomy in terms of decreased volumes with resulting clinical improvements following surgical ventricular restoration have been well documented. Improvements in ventricular function were assessed by the left ventricular ejection fraction which showed significant improvements. As detailed in the previous chapter, the technique of surgical ventricular restoration profoundly impacts the effective restoration of a near normal ventricular anatomy and function. The evolution in the surgical techniques has resulted in an evolutionary progress toward near normal ventricular restoration. The hemodynamics in the failing ventricle was discussed in Chap. 5. In this chapter, the hemodynamics following the various surgical techniques has been discussed. These hemodynamic studies are warranted in the surgically restored ventricle to assess its impact on ventricular function, which directly impacts morbidity and mortality.

The improvements in left ventricular volumes, left ventricular ejection fraction, and clinical improvements in NYHA class, quality of life, and decrease in the number of readmissions for heart failure all indicate overall hemodynamic improvement after surgical ventricular restoration. These improvements are based on decreases in left ventricular cavity radius which decreases wall stress based on Laplace's law.

However, the earlier technique of linear resection of the aneurismal tissue and repair resulted in a smaller ventricle with distorted geometry with incomplete scar tissue exclusion and inadequate revascularization of the contractile ischemic myocardium [1]. This resulted in increased mortality as compared to the geometric restoration or the endoventricular circular patch plasty (EVCPP). The systolic function as assessed by the left ventricular ejection fraction (LVEF) was also lesser than that of geometric restoration [1].

Even the EVCPP has been shown to result in a smaller spherical ventricle [2]. With increasing sphericity even in a nondilated ventricle, the mechanics of systolic and diastolic function, which are acutely dependent on ventricular torsion, are suboptimal [3, 4]. The left ventricular function is complex, and the ejection fraction is an inadequate measure of assessment. Therefore, the left ventricular function has been assessed by pressure–volume loops using conductance catheters [5–7].

Hemodynamics After Linear Repair at Rest and Following Exercise

Kawachi and coworkers studied patients subjected to the classical linear excision and repair [6]. At rest, they found a significant decrease in left ventricular volumes with increase in ejection fraction. The end-diastolic volume decreased postoperatively by 40.4%; the LVEF increased by 19%. The wall stress also decreased by 29.7% from the preoperative values.

The heart rate at rest before surgery and after surgery showed no significant difference. The

V R. Parachuri, S.M. Adhyapak, *Ventricular Geometry in Post-Myocardial Infarction Aneurysms*,
DOI 10.1007/978-1-4471-2861-8_9, © Springer-Verlag London 2012

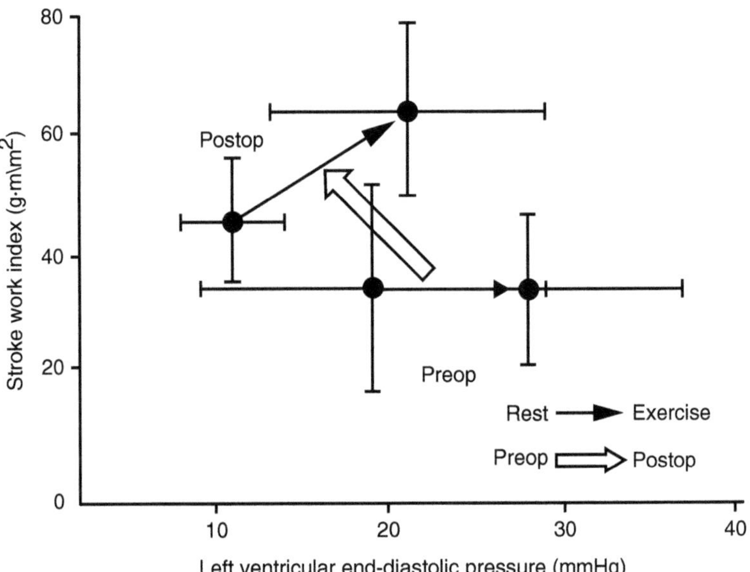

Fig. 9.1 Plots of the changes of SWI and LVEDP at rest and during exercise before and after the operation. After the operation, LVEDP at rest and during exercise slightly decreased compared with the preoperative value, whereas SWI slightly increased. These values shifted to the upper left portion of this figure (With permission from Kawachi et al. [6]. Copyright Elsevier)

heart rate during exercise was significantly higher than the rate at rest, increasing by 42% before surgery ($p<0.01$) and 44% ($p<0.01$) after surgery, respectively. The LV end-diastolic pressure (LVEDP) before and after surgery at rest were 19 ± 10and 11 ± 3 mmHg, respectively. The abnormally high preoperative value decreased after surgery, but the difference was not significant. During exercise, the LVEDP before and after surgery were 29 ± 10 and 21 ± 9 mmHg, respectively. Although the values were high, no significant difference was observed.

Cardiac index at rest was as low as 2.63 ± 0.9 L/min/m^2 before surgery but increased slightly to 3.10 ± 0.47 L/min/m^2 following surgery with no significant difference. Cardiac index during exercise was 3.53 ± 0.84 L/min/m^2 before surgery and 4.93 ± 1.00 L/min/m^2 after. Although the postoperative value was higher than the preoperative value, the difference was insignificant. The cardiac index during exercise increased significantly in comparison with that at rest, after linear repair.

Stroke volume index (SVI) at rest was 35 ± 6 mL/m^2 before the operation and 42 ± 9 mL/m^2 after surgery. During exercise, SVI was 36 ± 10 mL/m^2 before and 48 ± 10 mL/m^2 after surgery. The postoperative values were higher, but with no significant difference.

Stroke work index (SWI) at rest was 39 ± 17 g·m/m^2/beat before surgery and 49 ± 10 g·m/m^2/beat after. During exercise before and after surgery, SWI was 38 ± 13 and 65 ± 13 g·m/m^2/beat, respectively. The postoperative values were significantly higher than the preoperative values during exercise ($p<0.05$). In comparison with the SWI at rest, the SWI during exercise did not change significantly before and after the operation. Changes in SWI and LVEDP were shown by plotting the difference between the resting and exercise values for SWI (SWI) on the vertical axis and the difference between the resting and exercise values for LVEDP (LVEDP) on the horizontal axis. After SVR, all patients demonstrated increased SWI and LVEDP, indicating improvement. The changes before and after SVR in SWI and LVEDP at rest and during exercise were plotted in a graph. SWI was plotted on the vertical axis and LVEDP on the horizontal axis. After linear repair, LVEDP at rest and during exercise decreased compared with the preoperative values, whereas SWI showed an increase, the values shifting to the upper left portion of Fig. 9.1. This shift indicated improvement in the Frank–Starling curve.

These results are in contrast to those of Stephens and associates [8] who found that after aneurysmectomy, SWI did not change, but

LVEDP decreased at rest. In patients with severe symptoms and low EF at the contractile area of the LV, hemodynamic improvement was marked, whereas in patients with mild symptoms, the improvement was slight. In this study by Kawachi and coworkers, the cardiac index increased after SVR, although the increase was not statistically significant. After SVR, LVEDP showed a tendency to decrease, but no statistical difference was found.

There was a significant improvement in left ventricular volumes following linear repair which has a bearing on the wall stress which decreased significantly following linear repair. However, although the LVEDP decreased following surgery and cardiac index increased following surgery, both at rest and following exercise, the differences did not reach statistical significance. These changes were definitely discordant with earlier negative reports [8] on SVR for patients with left ventricular aneurysm and advanced heart failure. The significant improvements in stroke work index helped prove an improvement in the Frank–Starling curve.

Comparison of Hemodynamics Between Batista Surgery and SVR Done for Akinetic Versus Dyskinetic Left Ventricular Aneurysms

In order to establish the reasons for readmissions for heart failure in patients who have undergone heart reduction surgeries and surgical ventricular restoration, Artrip and coworkers studied the pressure–volume loops of patients subjected to ventricular reduction surgery—the Batista procedure—and patients with left ventricular aneurysms subjected to SVR by the EVCPP technique [9]. Laplace's law, which states the relationship between chamber diameter and wall stress, is cited as one of the physical principles underlying the potential benefits of volume reduction. Although it is true that a reduction of chamber radius will reduce wall stress for a given pressure, it is not obvious from this explanation alone that volume reduction will result in an increased pumping capacity of the heart. The analysis of reasons for failure of the Batista surgery revealed a potential limitation of this procedure: removing functioning (even weakened) myocardium, although reducing systolic wall stress and improving ejection fraction were associated with a deleterious effect on diastolic compliance that counteracted the beneficial effects on systolic wall stress. This might actually reduce net ventricular pumping capacity (indexed by the Frank–Starling relationship).

The SVR procedures differ conceptually from the Batista procedure in that instead of removing functioning myocardium, ventricular volume reduction is achieved through removing (or functionally excluding) stiff regions of akinetic scar or relatively more compliant dyskinetic scar. Although surgical treatment of dyskinetic scar (aneurysm) is considered accepted therapy for heart failure, there is less of a consensus regarding volume reduction through exclusion of akinetic wall segments and the physiological consequences of such procedures.

Theoretic Considerations

Mechanical pump properties of the normal left ventricle can be characterized by end-systolic and end-diastolic pressure–volume relationships (ESPVR and EDPVR, respectively), each of which quantifies the volume–capacitance of the chamber in the respective phase of the cardiac cycle. The ESPVR is relatively load independent and linear, with a slope (the end-systolic elastance [E_{es}]) that varies with myocardial contractility and a volume axis intercept (V_o) that varies with chamber size:

$$P_{es} = E_{es}(V_{es} - V_o)$$

where P_{es} and V_{es} are end-systolic pressure and volume, respectively. The EDPVR is exponential and commonly quantified by a stiffness coefficient (K) and a scaling factor (A) that vary with passive myocardial properties:

$$P_{ed} = A(e^{K(V_{ed} - V_o)} - 1)$$

where P_{ed} and V_{ed} are end-diastolic pressure (EDP) and end-diastolic volume, respectively. During a contraction, ventricular mechanical properties cycle between the end-diastolic and end-systolic properties described by these equations, which lead to the notion of the heart as a time-varying elastance that can be represented symbolically as a time-varying capacitive element [10].

In the event that myocardial properties differ from one region to the next, global ventricular properties can be represented by the interaction between two capacitive elements, each with its own pressure–volume characteristics. The effective pressure–volume relations of each region will depend on the time-varying material properties of that region and the proportion of total ventricular mass having those properties. Because at each instant of the cardiac cycle both portions of the chamber are exposed to the same pressure, the pressure–volume properties of the composite ventricle are determined by adding volumes at each pressure, as shown for the ESPVRs and EDPVRs.

After a transmural myocardial infarction, the material properties of the affected region can be varied. In some instances, the infarcted myocardium can be stiff, resulting in an akinetic region with a steep pressure–volume relationship. Alternatively, the infarcted region can be compliant, resulting in a dyskinetic scar with a shallow pressure–volume relationship.

To illustrate the three major forms of ventricular reduction surgery, Batista surgery, excision of dyskinetic and akinetic aneurysms, 20% of the left ventricle was given properties of either weak but contracting muscle, an akinetic scar, or a dyskinetic scar. The remainder of the heart was composed of contracting muscle, and the composite properties of the ventricles (in terms of ESPVR and EDPVR) for the starting heart failure state were the same for all three conditions. The properties of the akinetic scar and dyskinetic scar were each described by a time-invariant pressure–volume relationship with the equation for the EDPVR and similar parameters, except for a stiffness coefficient set to ten times the normal value for the akinetic scar and one half the normal value for the dyskinetic scar.

Maximum total work at any EDP was quantified by the maximum pressure–volume area (PVA_{max}), which is the area confined within the ESPVR and EDPVR between V_0 and the end-diastolic volume at the EDP of interest.

When weak but contracting muscle is removed (Batista procedure), the EDPVR is shifted more to the left than is the ESPVR. This reduces the area between the ESPVR and EDPVR compared with the original heart, which will have detrimental effects on overall pump properties. When stiff, noncontracting myocardium (akinetic) is removed (or excluded), the EDPVR and ESPVR shift by similar amounts at all pressures. Thus, the area between the ESPVR and EDPVR is relatively unchanged from the original state.

When compliant dyskinetic myocardium is removed, the effect on the pressure–volume relationship is highly pressure dependent. For the EDPVR, which resides at lower pressures, there is less of a leftward shift than for the ESPVR at higher pressures. As a result, the curvilinearity of this relationship is affected, and there is a significant increase in the area between the ESPVR and EDPVR.

Removal or exclusion of any segment of ventricular wall (regardless of function) resulted in a leftward shift of the ESPVR (i.e., decrease in the V_0 value), but changes in the slope (i.e., increase in the E_{es} value) depended on the type of muscle being resected. The E_{es} values obtained were greatest after removal of dyskinetic scar and increased after removal of contracting myocardium but were nearly identical to the baseline heart failure state after removal of akinetic scar. Ventricular diastolic stiffness was also increased after removal of dyskinetic scar or contracting myocardium but was approximately unchanged after removal of akinetic myocardium.

The relationship between PVA_{max} (an index of total ventricular work) and EDP provides a load-independent assessment of global ventricular pump function. As suggested above by the description of differential shifts in ESPVRs and EDPVRs, removal of contracting myocardium (Batista procedure) shifts the curve downward from baseline, whereas removal of akinetic scar does not significantly change the curve from baseline. However, removal of dyskinetic scar shifts the curve upward from baseline, suggesting improved overall pumping capacity.

Removing functioning myocardium reduces peak wall stress–pressure relationships but at the expense of increased diastolic wall stiffness, with a net reduction in overall ventricular pump function. Removal of contracting myocardium or dyskinetic scar significantly increased E_{es}, whereas removal of an akinetic myocardial segment had little effect on this value. Removal of a dyskinetic scar or contracting myocardium resulted in significantly stiffer chambers, whereas removal of an akinetic myocardial segment had little effect on this relationship other than to shift it leftward.

The PVA_{max}-EDP relationship provides an afterload-independent assessment of pump function and indexes the area between the end-diastolic pressure–volume and end-systolic pressure–volume relationships. The results demonstrated a beneficial effect of removing dyskinetic scar, an equivocal effect of removing akinetic myocardium, and a negative effect of removing contracting myocardium on overall ventricular pump function. Removal of contracting myocardium (Batista) affected diastolic properties more than systolic properties, resulting in a net decrease in pump function. In contrast, removal of compliant, dyskinetic infarcted tissue more significantly affected systolic properties than diastolic properties, resulting in increased pump function. Finally, removal or exclusion of stiff, akinetic infarcted tissue equally affected systolic and diastolic properties, resulting in no significant change in pump function.

Hemodynamics Following EVCPP

Tulner and colleagues [5] studied ten patients before and immediately after EVCPP by pressure–volume loops. The fundamental question to be addressed was whether, in aggregate, the changes in hemodynamics and ventricular properties induced by surgically reducing the size of the heart were favorable or unfavorable. Since pressure–volume analysis provides the most comprehensive means of assessing ventricular contractile properties, and the most rigorous means of measuring these relations in the clinical setting is with the conductance catheter, they studied the hemodynamics before and after EVCPP by conductance catheter studies.

The increase in EF following SVR provides support for the assertion of improved left ventricular pump function, although it is known that reduction of EDV without an increase in EF would result in inadequate SV. However, with other interventions like valve replacements resulting in amelioration of native valve regurgitations, an increase of EF results from an increase in SV with little change in EDV. In contrast, the increase in EF observed with SVR results from a decrease in EDV with little change in SV. The reduced peak and end-systolic left ventricular pressures (decreased afterload) and marked elevation of end-diastolic pressure (increased preload) with no increase in SV observed after SVR could actually imply reduced pumping capability.

With ESV_{80} that is the ESV at a pressure of 80 mmHg, as detailed by Tulner and colleagues used to index the ESPVR position, SVR resulted in an approximately 54 mL leftward shift of the average ESPVR with only a small increase in the slope of the ESPVR (Fig. 9.2). This compares with a leftward EDPVR shift of approximately 83 mL using EDV_{14} that is the EDV at a pressure of 14 mmHg, to index the EDPVR position; chamber stiffness is also increased, which further accentuates the impact on diastolic properties. Thus, the magnitude of the leftward shift of the EDPVR is approximately 30 mL greater than that of the ESPVR.

This, in turn, signifies a reduction of overall pump function as revealed by the overall pump function curves, which show isovolumic pressure–volume area (PVA_{ISO}) as a function of end-diastolic pressure. PVA_{ISO} is the area on the pressure–volume diagram of the triangular region contained between the EDPVR and ESPVR at each EDV. At increasing EDVs, end-diastolic pressure increases according to the EDPVR, and PVA_{ISO} increases according to the relative positions of the EDPVR and ESPVR. PVA_{ISO} is a measure of the total possible mechanical energy the

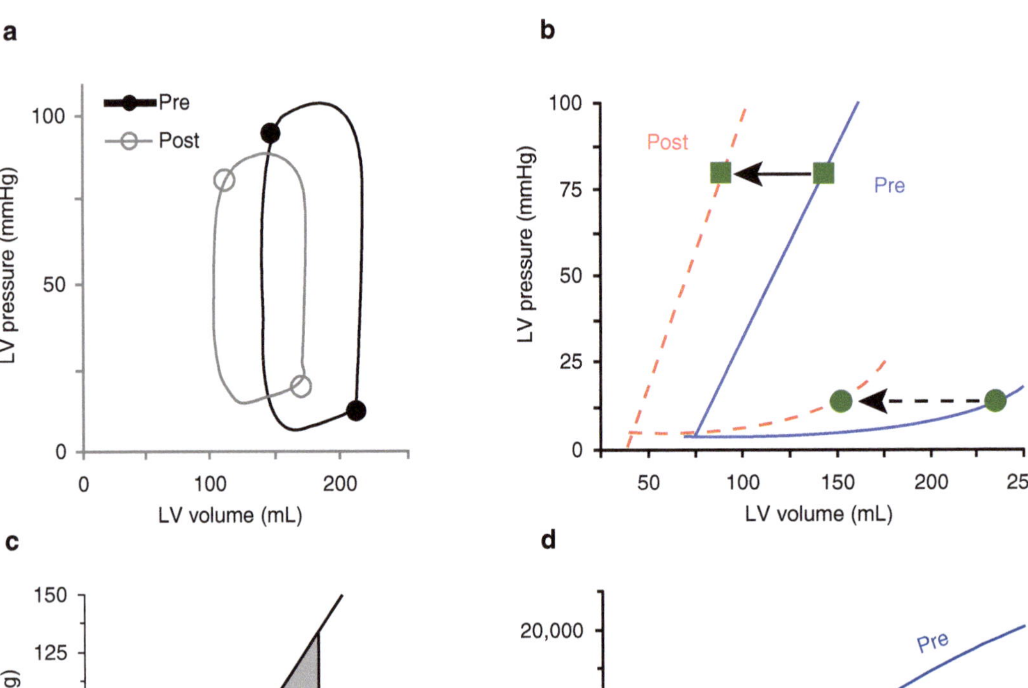

Fig. 9.2 (**a**) Reproduction of the average pressure–volume loops obtained by Tulner and associates. (**b**) End-systolic and end-diastolic pressure–volume relations were constructed from the average results of Tulner and associates. Preoperative (*Pre*) relations are shown by *solid lines*, and postoperative (*Post*) relations are shown by *dashed lines*. Volumes at a systolic pressure of 80 mmHg are shown by *squares*, and diastolic volumes at a pressure of 14 mmHg are shown by *circles*. *Arrows* show respective shift of ESPVR (*solid lined arrow*) and EDPVR (*dashed line arrow*), respectively. The shift of EDPVR is greater than the shift of the ESPVR. (**c**) Demonstration of how isovolumic pressure–volume area (PVA_{ISO}) is calculated from the pressure–volume diagram. One value for PVA_{ISO} can be obtained for each end-diastolic pressure–volume point. The end-diastolic pressure–volume point (EDP) for this example is shown by the *solid red circle*. (**d**) The relationship between PVA_{ISO} and EDP is constructed from the preoperative and postoperative EDPVRs and ESPVRs of panel (**b**). The postoperative relationship is lower than the preoperative relation, signifying a reduction in the maximum work capacity of the heart (With permission from Burkhoff et al. [11]. Copyright Elsevier)

ventricle can generate at the specified preload pressure and thus provides an afterload-independent measure of the pumping capability of the heart. The relationship between end-diastolic pressure and PVA_{ISO} is shifted downward after SVR, indicating that at any given filling pressure the heart is capable of less work than before the procedure. In aggregate, the changes in the pressure–volume loops and pressure–volume relationships resemble those observed in diastolic heart failure. However, this interpretation must be tempered by the fact that the heart is now working at more physiological volumes. They also demonstrated improved mechanical efficiency following SVR. Mechanical efficiency (ME) was calculated as the ratio of stroke work and pressure–volume area: ME=SW/PVA (Fig. 9.2).

Acutely after SVR, there were significant decreases in left ventricular volumes in diastole and systole, increases in ejection fraction, improvements in mechanical efficiency, improvements in mechanical dyssynchrony, with leftward shifts of both the end-systolic pressure volume curve and the end-diastolic pressure–volume curve, an unchanged or decreased stroke volume, increased diastolic stiffness of the ventricle, and increased end-diastolic pressure. However, the maintained stroke work that was obtained at a higher end-diastolic pressure was a negative aspect because, even with an unchanged Frank–Starling curve, this indicates that the possibility to increase stroke work (or cardiac output) via this mechanism is limited. Thus, overall in this study, it was found that SVR improved systolic ventricular function at the expense of worsening diastolic function, which theoretically implied a negative overall pump function of the heart.

However, these results could be cofounded by the acute effects of surgery, mainly edema, use of inotropes and vasodilators in the acute setting. Hence, these studies were repeated by the same authors [12] on patients subjected to EVCPP, 6 months following surgery.

At 6 months following EVCPP, all patients were alive and clinically in improved condition: New York Heart Association class improved from 3.3±0.5 to 1.4±0.7, quality-of-life score improved from 46±22 to 15±15, and 6-min hall-walk test improved from 302±123 to 444±78 m (all $p<0.01$). Hemodynamic data showed improved cardiac output (4.8±1.4 to 5.6±1.1 L/min), stroke work (6.5±1.9 to 7.1±1.4 mmHg L; $p=0.05$), and left ventricular ejection fraction (36%±10% to 46%±10%; $p<0.001$). Left ventricular surgical remodeling was sustained at 6 months: end-diastolic volume decreased from 246±70 to 180±48 mL and end-systolic volume from 173±77 to 103±40 mL (both $p<0.001$). Left ventricular dyssynchrony decreased from 29%±6% to 26%±3% ($p<0.001$), and ineffective internal flow fraction decreased from 58%±30% to 42%±18% ($p<0.005$). Early relaxation (Tau, minimal rate of pressure change) was unchanged, but diastolic stiffness constant increased from 0.012±0.003 to 0.023±0.007 mL^{-1} ($p<0.001$). Improved systolic function and unchanged early diastolic function with impaired passive diastolic properties were noted at 6 months following EVCPP. Clinical improvement, supported by decreased New York Heart Association class, improved quality-of-life score, and improved 6-min hall-walk test might be related to improved systolic function, reduced mechanical dyssynchrony, and reduced wall stress.

The persistence of diastolic dysfunction at 6 months following surgery cannot be attributed to cardiac wall edema and other acute effects of surgery. These findings should be interpreted in the light of Artrip's findings. Therefore, it is necessary to quantify the material properties of the scarred area or aneurismal area as akinetic or dyskinetic. The standard approach would be by MRI studies as echocardiographic studies for material property delineation are less specific.

The second factor responsible for the diastolic dysfunction could be the residual volume of the left ventricle following surgery. Tulner and coworkers used a balloon measuring device of 55 mL/BSA. This may not be a standard residual cavity, as seen by Menicanti and coworkers [13]. They adjusted the volume of the measuring device according to the preoperative left ventricular volumes. Di Donato and coworkers [14] found that those patients with greater end-diastolic volumes at baseline had greater reductions of volumes after SVR, but demonstrated redilatation at long term (6 months to 1 year) following surgery. Those patients with larger residual ventricular cavities following SVR also demonstrated greater degrees of redilatation of up to 15% at long term following surgery [2]. Serenella Castellvecchio [15] found that irrespective of preoperative end-diastolic volume, the left ventricles with a more conical apex (conicity index <1) had worse diastolic dysfunction as compared with equally dilated left ventricular cavities which were mainly dilated at the apical level, that is more spherical ventricles (conicity index >1). Also, if reductions of end-diastolic volumes were lesser, leaving a larger residual ventricle, or if the reductions of end-diastolic volumes were higher, leaving a small residual ventricular cavity, diastolic dysfunction would ensue. Although, this had no effect on mortality, the patients with diastolic dysfunction were more likely to be in NYHA classes III and IV, with resulting increased readmissions for heart failure. This again brings us back to the surgical technique of restoration of the aneurismal left ventricle. The technique of EVCPP, although helps realigning the oblique myocardial fibers from a diseased horizontal orientation to a more oblique orientation, still results in a smaller but more spherical ventricle which is subject to late adverse remodeling [2].

Therefore, there is a need to study the hemodynamics following modified geometric repairs which are more oriented to restoration of ventricular shape than ventricular volume alone. Data on hemodynamics after modified geometric repair are lacking.

Ventricular Efficiency

Cardiac function is balanced upon optimal filling and ejection into the arterial system. There has been a lot of interest in the interaction between the heart and the vasculature, particularly with regard to the determinants of cardiac work or flow output and determinants of myocardial oxygen consumption. The ratio of ventricular stroke work (SW) to ventricular oxygen consumption is defined as ventricular efficiency. The E_{es} is defined as the slope of the end-systolic pressure–volume relationship, and ventricular afterload is defined as E_a. Therefore, in the normal heart, the SW is maximum when $E_a = E_{es}$. Also, the afterload that results in the greatest efficiency is always less than that which provides maximum SW. In heart failure, the SW and efficiency are more sensitive to changes in afterload than in the normal heart. The ventricular efficiency and end-diastolic volume have a sigmoidal relation which reaches its maximum at end-diastolic volumes above the upper limits of the physiological range.

Tanoue and coworkers [7] have studied ventricular energetic in large anterior left ventricular aneurysms following EVCPP. End-systolic elastance (E_{es}) increased after the procedure (from 1.15±0.60 to 1.86±0.84 mmHg m^2 mL^{-1}, $p<0.01$), resulting in an improvement in ventriculoarterial coupling (E_a/E_{es}) (from 2.94±1.11 to 1.64±0.49, $p<0.01$), even though E_a did not substantially change (from 2.96±0.78 to 2.74±0.55 mmHg m^2 mL^{-1}, $p=0.4$). Ventricular stroke work/pressure volume area (SW/PVA) efficiency was also improved (from 0.426±0.110 to 0.559±0.082, $p<0.01$.). The contractility (E_{es}) improved; afterload (E_a) did not change. These changes resulted in an improvement in the ventricular efficiency (E_a/E_{es} and SW/PVA). Following EVCPP there was improvement in ventricular efficiency, due to improvements in contractility. The afterload remained unchanged from preoperative values, indicating the need for afterload reducing agents following surgery. The conventional hemodynamic variables (heart rate, pulmonary capillary wedge pressure, mean blood pressure, and cardiac index) did not change after EVCPP in this study. The significant changes were limited to the load-independent variables.

Ventriculoarterial coupling has been studied in patients who underwent the EVCPP procedure by Fantini and colleagues [16]. They reported that ventriculoarterial coupling improved after the surgery mainly because of the decrease in E_a. After surgery, they found marked reductions in left ventricular volumes and significant increases in ejection fraction, without changes in mean SVI and stroke work. End-diastolic pressure decreased slightly; end-systolic pressure decreased. Pulmonary vascular resistance index (PVRI) did not show a significant reduction.

The changes in E_a were related both to its preoperative values and to the postoperative improvement in the ejection fraction the greatest reduction in E_a occurred in patients with higher preoperative values of E_a ($r=0.84$, $p<0.0001$) and in those patients with a greater postoperative increase in ejection fraction ($r=0.67$, $p<0.001$). E_{max} and chamber mechanical efficiency increased significantly after surgery. The marked postoperative reduction in EDVI associated with a decrease in end-diastolic pressure indicated a decrease in left ventricular preload. The lack of postoperative changes in stroke work and stroke volume, in the presence of improved ejection fraction and decreased E_a, further confirms the role played by left ventricular volume decrease. Left ventricular pump function improved after surgery, following Starling's law (maintenance of the same stroke work with a decreased preload). Further evidence of this improvement is the marked increase in mechanical efficiency and the mild increase in E_{max}. The higher E_{max} shown by the restored left ventricle appeared to be a result of the sharp reduction in ESVI. The ratio between arterial and ventricular elastance decreased after surgery, mainly because of the greater decrease in arterial elastance than the lesser increase in ventricular elastance. The decrease in arterial elastance appeared to be related mainly to a reduction in end-systolic pressure. In the absence of changes in heart rate, stroke volume, and peripheral vascular resistance—and assuming only minor changes in inotropic state and in the structural characteristics of the arterial wall—these changes mainly reflect loading sequence changes induced by the patch plasty reconstruction.

Improvements in Mechanical Synchrony Following EVCPP

Studies are lacking in reporting improvements in mechanical synchrony following linear plication and repair for left ventricular aneurysms. Di Donato et al. [17] have studied patients with left ventricular aneurysms following EVCPP.

Regional differences improved after restoration, because SVR made almost all regions develop more uniform endocardial motion that reached its maximum extent at end-systolic phase. Such uniformity contributed ejection without wasting energy, thereby defining mechanical resynchronization.

Analysis of pressure/volume loops provided a more sensitive means of examining regional components of synchrony and uniformity, because they defined contraction of given segments toward global LV performance. The area enclosed by each loop over the entire course of the cardiac cycle reflects the net mechanical work of the myocardial segment. Although LV pressure reflects the time course of contraction of LV mass, local segment length provides focus and reflects the time course of the contraction of the ischemic/scarred segment and how it interacts with adjacent normal myocardium.

Before surgery, most P/L loops showed abnormalities in morphology, size, and orientation. The most common observed abnormalities were early shortening and early relaxation, with markedly reduced effective work. Early shortening occurs because of the unloading effect of dyskinetic myocardium in series, which acts as an elastic slack element during the isovolumic phase of contraction. Right-oriented CW loops were also observed at the anteroapical regions preoperatively. This type of loop abnormality means the loss of all contractile properties. Paradoxical systolic expansion means absence of force development and stretching by adjacent normal fibers. Early shortening and early lengthening are experimentally reproducible by connecting weak and strong myocardium in series. Thus, within one cardiac cycle, regional P/L loops move in an opposite direction and asynchronously, giving each region a different contribution to global ejection.

Postoperatively, an almost complete reversal of P/L loops abnormalities occurred in regions remote from anterior scar. Most loops in the inferior regions reverted to normal orientation and shape, with steeper isometric phases and increased area, reflecting an increased effective work and more synchronous ejection.

This confirms that relieving the abnormal tension by excluding the scar and reducing the volume allows SVR to improve overall mechanical performance by increasing effective work of each single loop. Normalization of most regional P/L loops became transcribed into marked improvement in isovolumic phases of the global P/V loops and increased mechanical efficiency. The reduction of dyssynchrony during the relaxation phase likely explains the improvement in global LV diastolic function, as evidenced by the improvement in Tau and PVR.

Acute hemodynamic improvement induced by SVR depends on a complex interplay of changes in LV geometry and shape, loading conditions, and stress distribution within the LV wall. In fact, this surgical intervention includes revascularization, reduction of mitral regurgitation, and exclusion of the scar, and all these procedures may be beneficial to pump function improvement by relieving ischemia and reducing volume overload and remodeling. Consequently, the effects of SVR are complex, and the observed mechanical resynchronization can be hypothesized to contribute to the postoperative improvement in function. Ventricular restoration by SVR is a fixed geometric event that changes many hemodynamic determinants of cardiac function, so that the effective role of mechanical resynchronization cannot be quantified. These induced anatomic changes are not reversible like electrical resynchronization induced by biventricular pacing, and so cannot be compared with those obtained after electrical stimulation.

MRI Hemodynamic Studies Following EVCPP

Following EVCPP, the end-diastolic volume and end-systolic volumes decreased significantly, with increases in stroke volume and ejection fraction [18]. The circumferential strain increased in the remote myocardium by 19% (7.3 ± 2.4 to 8.7 ± 2.3, $p < 0.05$). There was no change in circumferential strain in the adjacent or repaired regions. This increase was not significant late after surgery (8.9 ± 2.1). The meridonial strain at the repair site showed lengthening immediately following surgery and a trend toward shortening late after surgery. There were no significant changes in the adjacent and remote regions. An increasing gradient in the radial strain between repair and remote regions was seen at preoperative, postoperative, and at long term after surgery ($p < 0.05$). The circumferential–longitudinal shear was unchanged. The maximum principle strain increased immediately after surgery and remained so at follow-up (10 ± 4 to 15 ± 2 to 14 ± 5, $p < 0.005$). There was no significant difference in minimum principle strain. Phi, the angle between the circumferential direction and the minimum principle strain, changed from before surgery to late after surgery, from -21 ± 16 to $-10 \pm 22°$ ($p < 0.005$) becoming globally more circumferential. However, regionally, Phi became oriented more longitudinally and directly correlated with the distance from the surgical patch. This indicated that following EVCPP, reverse remodeling occurred which was coupled with improvements in intramyocardial mechanics predominantly in the remote myocardium at 1 year.

Although torsion increased from base to apex following surgery, the mean global torsion did not differ significantly from preoperative values (0.16 ± 0.1 vs. 0.15 ± 0.06, $p = 0.56$).

Evaluation of the Restored Ventricular Geometry

A global prolate ellipse was fit to each left ventricle in the two chamber and four chamber view using the major and minor axes at the base. Secondly, an apical prolate ellipse was fit to a section positioned at two-thirds of the major axis to more appropriately define the newly restored apical geometry. Finally, the ratio of the apical/global minor axis ellipses in each projection characterizing the agreement or the amount of heterogeneity between the two prolate ellipses was examined (Fig. 9.3). As the ratio approached unity, the apical ellipse approximated the global ellipse, implying that the apical shape precisely tracked the global geometry. In normal individuals, there is a high degree of agreement between the global ellipse and apical ellipse regardless of the point of measurement, indicating preservation of basal to apical symmetry. In contrast, patients with ischemic cardiomyopathy deviate far from normal as one interrogates more apically, than toward the base. Following EVCPP, the measured apical/global heterogeneity geometry index moved leftward and down approaching that of normals, revealing a strong trend toward normalization of ventricular geometry with EVCPP. But, despite normalization of LV

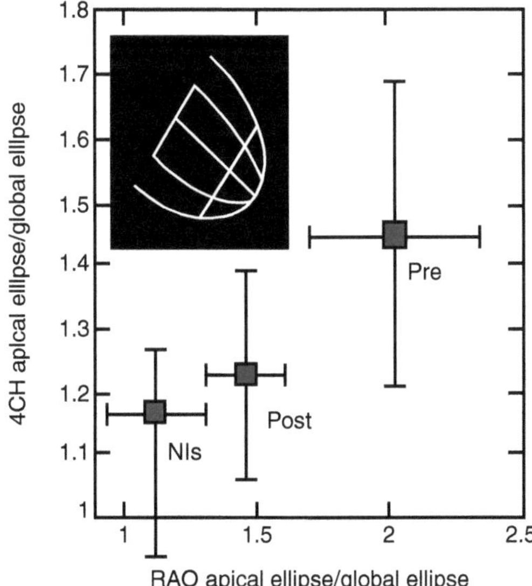

Fig. 9.3 Quantification of left ventricular shape following EVCPP by the global ellipse and apical ellipse method on MRI (With permission from Open Magn Reson. 2009;2:33–45. Open Access Journal)

volume by EVCPP, the geometry was still not ideal. Examination revealed that an apical truncation process was in effect. Simple recreation of the Fontan suture and surgical exclusion of the apex perpendicular to the long axis of the LV result in a "snub nose" LV defeating significant gains appropriated from a reduction in Laplacian stress [19] (Fig. 9.3).

Based on the RESTORE group analysis, the EF increased from 29.6 ± 11% to 39.5 ± 12.3% after surgery. In terms of simulated energy model parameters, this corresponded to a mean decrease in basal energy (BE) of 26% and a mean increase in SW of 12% with net work decreasing by only 9%. Compared to normal individuals, these values are still elevated. In normal individuals, BE is approximately one-third of SW, and by matching the EF values of the patients prior to surgery, the mean ratio of BE/SW was 1.23, representing a reversal of energy distribution as compared to normals. Following surgery, the BE/SW ratio decreased to 0.8, representing a progression toward normalization, but clearly remaining in the abnormal range. This analysis also reflects the suboptimal restoration of the ventricular ellipse by EVCPP, which was clearly seen to be truncated at the apex.

Hemodynamic Changes Following EVLPP in Comparison with EVCPP

Although hemodynamic studies are lacking after modified geometric ventricular restoration techniques, Parachuri and coworkers [20] have compared the results of EVLPP and EVCPP. They used echocardiographic quantification of left ventricular volumes and left ventricular ejection fraction to evaluate the relationship of the percent decrease in end-diastolic volume to the percent increase in left ventricular ejection fraction and percent decrease in end-diastolic volume to percent change in stroke volume following EVLPP and compare these changes with EVCPP. Linear endoventricular patch plasty resulted in a decrease in end-diastolic volume of 40.2 mL (95% confidence interval (CI): 33.6, 46.7) and stroke volume of 10.0 mL (95% CI: 6.6, 13.5) and increase in ejection fraction of 6.7% (95% CI: 5.5, 7.9). There was a further 14% decrease in EDV and SV (30%) at 2 years with increase in EF (20%). There was a persistent significant improvement in sphericity index.

Relationship of Percent Change in EDV to Percent Change in SV

Following EVCPP when the percent change in EDVI was compared with percent changes in SVI, the relationship was J shaped (Fig. 8.8). The changes in SVI were not proportional to the EDVI especially for larger decreases in EDVI. This relates to the geometry and size of the noncontractile area in the ventricle, which corresponds to the circular/oval endoventricular patch. When the EDVI is reduced by a large magnitude, with an akinetic circular endoventricular patch, the changes in SVI are not proportional to the changes in EDVI. This also relates to the anatomical substrate of the restored left ventricle, where improvements were only seen in the inferior wall curvature with no change in the anterior wall.

The resultant surgically restored ventricle remained spherical albeit with a reduced radius. With EVCPP, the oblique fibers continue to have a slightly horizontal orientation with resultant ineffective systolic shortening reflected by the SVI, and contributing to late re-remodeling especially in patients with large preoperative EDVI. With EVLPP, the change in SVI had a significant linear relationship with change in EDVI across all magnitudes of EDVI reduction (Fig. 9.4 a, b). This relationship was persistent even 2 years after surgery. Hence, by decreasing the akinetic area to <25% of the ventricular surface area and by configuring its geometry to a linear geometry, the realignment of the anterior and anterolateral ventricular walls is better accomplished, resulting in a near physiological ellipsoid ventricular geometry, while maintaining physiological interactions between the ventricular volumes with persistent late reverse remodeling.

Relationship of Percent Changes in EDV to Percent Changes in EF

In the normal heart, during systole, the percent decrease in LV diameter is proportional to the percent increase in EF [20]. This is true as long as the ventricle is ellipsoid, with intact helical fiber orientation. The EF decreases when percent decrease in LV diameter approaches the value of percent decrease in ventricular length from base to apex during ventricular contraction, that is when the ventricular configuration becomes spherical with dilatation. The increase in EF with decreases in EDV has been documented with all techniques of SVR. Following EVCPP, the relationship of percent change in EDVI and percent change in EF was curvilinear (Fig. 9.5). The decreases in EDVI were not inversely proportional to increases in the EF across all magnitudes of EDVI decrease. With EVLPP, there was a significant inverse linear relationship between EDVI and EF across all magnitudes of EDVI decrease early after surgery.

This linearity between EDVI and EF was not present 2 years after EVLPP. The EF has several limitations in assessing LV pump function following SVR. The clinical improvements are far better than the magnitude of increase in EF. This discrepancy could have its origin in the fact that SVR does not uniformly result in an increase in SV. This paradox has been explained below. Hence, the linear relationship of the EDVI with SVI which persisted late after EVLPP serves as a marker of physiological ellipsoid LV geometry.

Effect of Ventricular Dilatation on the SV in the Failing Ventricle Extension of the Frank–Starling Mechanism in the Failing Heart

The geometrical determinants of cardiac SV have been evaluated on the basis of mathematical models of the left ventricle [21].

It has been found that despite increasing wall stress, the SV generally increases with increasing anatomical cardiac size, reaching a maximum beyond which it decreases. On the basis of a model of a thick walled sphere representing the LV, SV relations have been computed for three different types of chronic ventricular enlargement. The three models are that of concentric hypertrophy, eccentric hypertrophy, and predominant increases of ventricular volume without hypertrophy. In all three models, the SV increases correlated only with increasing ventricular size up to a certain size, and decreased as the size was increased further. Thus, it was hypothesized that the SV can be augmented with increasing ventricular size, under constant contractility despite decreasing ejection fractions [21]. Here, the slope of the curve describing the relation between SV and anatomical ventricular size was flattened, and the maximum of the curve was shifted toward smaller EDVs in the presence of reduced contractility, distensibility, or after loss of contractile tissue. Human studies of heart failure have shown that pumping failure occurs when the ventricular operating point has reached the maximum, so that compensation by increase in ventricular size has been exhausted [21–24]. This hypothesis is an extension of the Frank–Starling mechanism operating in ischemic cardiomyopathy, where the SV increases with increasing EDV beyond the normal EDV limit, with decreasing contractility and decreasing EF. This

Fig. 9.4 Relationship of EDVI and SVI immediately after EVLPP (**a**) and at 2 years follow-up (**b**)

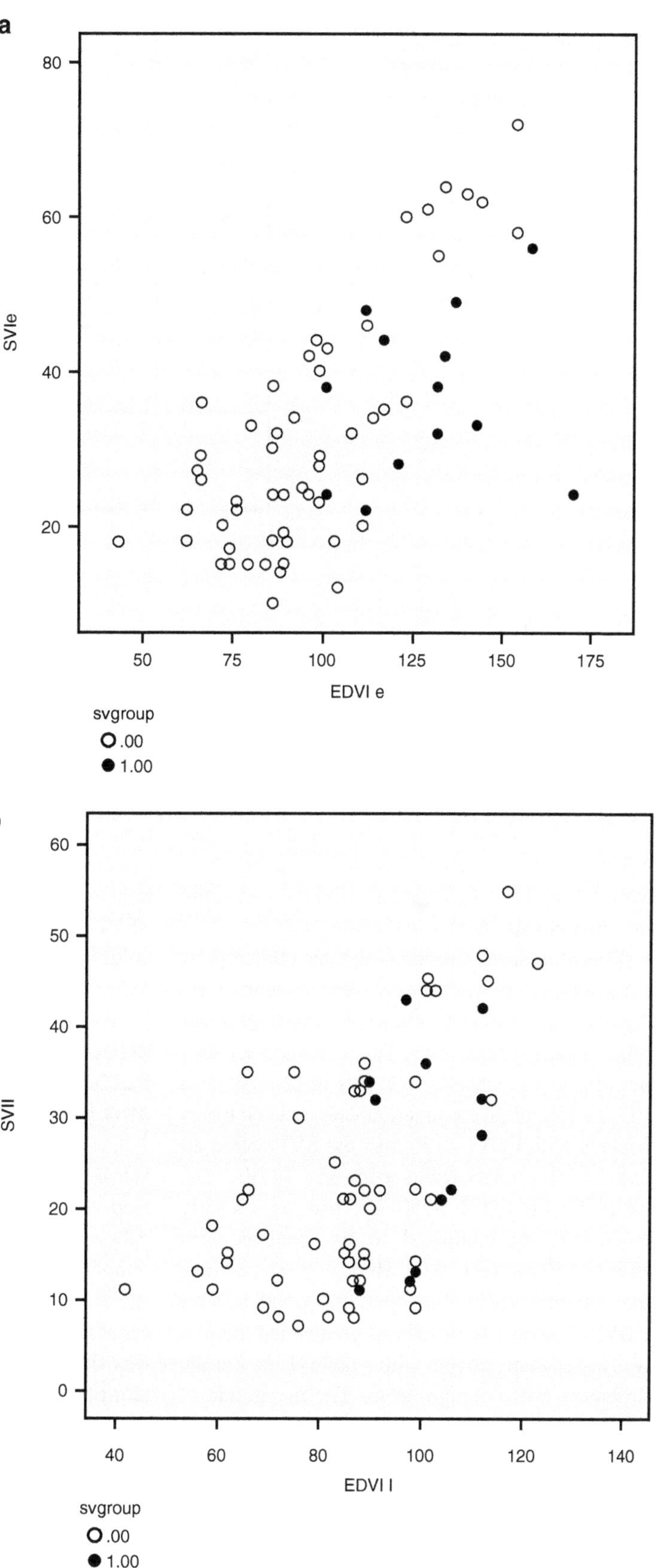

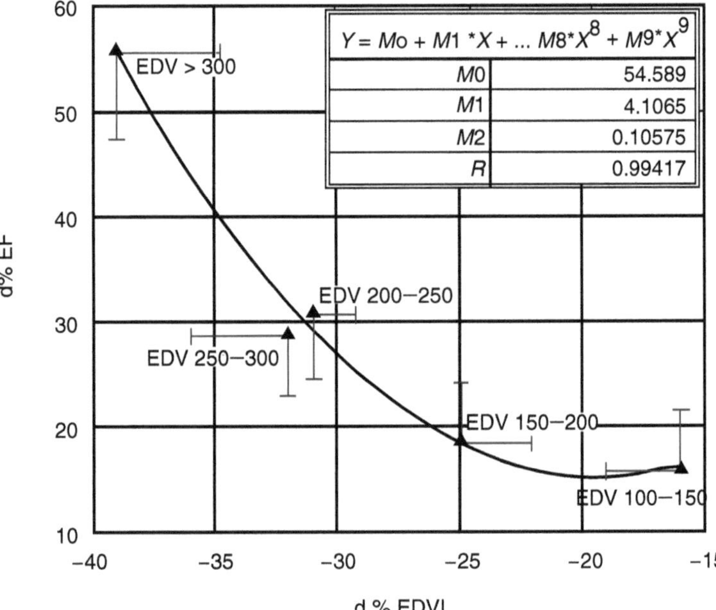

Fig. 9.5 Relationship of percent reduction on EDVI and percent increase in EF following EVCPP (With permission from Adhyapak et al. [20]. Copyright Elsevier)

mechanism is explained by the increased sensitivity of the calcium channels in the existing contractile myocardium [23, 24]. When a certain magnitude of EDV is reached, that is the point of maximal compensation of the SV to increases in EDV, the SV begins to decline. This decline in SV is related to the degree of LV dilatation only and not related to the presence of compensatory remodeling. At this point, the sensitivity of calcium channels in the contractile myocardium also begins to decline.

This hypothesis has been validated clinically by Parachuri and coworkers. In these patients, only the EDVI and EF were related in significant linear relationships with the SVI. The SVI increased proportionally to increases in EDVI in patients with EDVI ≤ 150 mL in conjunction with reduced EF. In patients with EDVI ≥150 mL, the SVI decreased and had no relationship with the EDVI. The patients with EDVI >150 mL had significantly larger LVs as compared to the patients with EDVI < 150 mL (Fig. 9.6). Thus, in these patients, the maximal ventricular operating point was an EDVI > 150 mL. Their EF was greater and the SVI was lesser than patients with smaller LVs, but the difference was not significant. The magnitude of EDVI at the maximal ventricular operating point in relation to increments in SVI for each individual patient, beyond which the SVI declines, may vary.

In the normal heart under various physiological loading conditions, the ESVI bears a significant linear relationship to the EF [26]. In these patients, there was no significant relationship between ESVI and SVI and ESVI and EF. The reason for this phenomenon could be that in the course of remodeling, the dilated LV attempts to compensate by decreasing its ESVI to maintain an effective cardiac output, and hence the ESVI may not be significantly related to its stroke volume or EF.

Effect of Geometric Remodeling Patterns on the SV: Effect of Preload and Afterload

While studying the effect of preload and afterload on the SV, the two geometric remodeling patterns of eccentric hypertrophy and concentric remodeling were studied. The pattern of eccentric hypertrophy was the substrate for preload excess, and the pattern of concentric remodeling was the substrate for afterload excess. The pattern of eccentric hypertrophy most likely reflects the increase in venous return that, in the absence of an increase in peripheral needs, depends on an increase in circulatory mass, which in turn

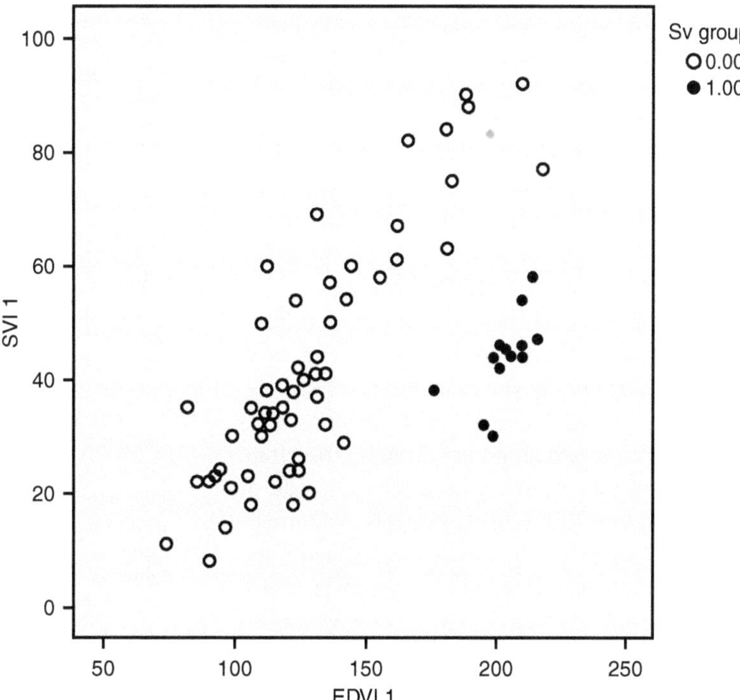

Fig. 9.6 Relationship of EDVI and SVI at baseline and following EVLPP. Marker 0 (*clear circles*) = Patients who demonstrated increase in SV with increases in EDV at baseline, Marker 1 (*black circles*) = Patients who did not demonstrate an increase in SV at baseline with increases in EDV (With permission from Adhyapak and Parachuri [25]. Copyright Elsevier)

depends on water and sodium retention. In other words, eccentric remodeling identifies a "backward heart failure" secondary to the increase in filling pressure with pulmonary congestion. This factor is rarely taken into account when pressure/volume loops of ventricles with different geometries are compared. In this study, the patients with eccentric hypertrophy had significantly greater LV EDVI and ESVI with lesser EF, signifying greater degrees of LV dilatation than patients with concentric remodeling. The EF was better preserved in the concentric remodeling group. The presence of both concentric remodeling and eccentric hypertrophy had no significant effect on the SVI.

In these patients, where there was no significant left ventricular diastolic dysfunction, and no significant mitral regurgitation to confound the reductions in SVI following SVR, the model studies of Gulch and coworkers [21], where perturbations in the preload or afterload seen as representative forms of ventricular remodeling patterns of eccentric hypertrophy and concentric remodeling, have no effect on the SVI in heart failure, and beyond the maximal ventricular operating point, only increases in EDVI cause decreases in SV [21–23] stand clinically validated.

The Relationship of EDV and SV: Frank–Starling Relationship in the Surgically Restored Ventricle

Following SVR by the technique of EVLPP, although there was a decrease in SV by 10 mL, there were significant clinical improvements. A 31% decrease in ESVI was found following surgery with an additional decrease of 5.4% in ESVI at 2 years, signifying persistent reverse remodeling with absence of re-remodeling. In these patients, the occurrence of left ventricular diastolic dysfunction was seen only in those with EDVI > 250 mL. Following SVR, the diastolic dysfunction improved from grade III to grade I. The sphericity index also showed significant improvements following surgery and demonstrated further significant improvements at 2 years.

Although the SVI either decreased from baseline in patients with marker = 0 or remained the same in patients with marker = 1, this decrease in

SVI should not be noted as a marker of impaired LV function. The decreases in EDVI following SVR lead to decreases in SVI from baseline in patients with increased baseline SVI, and in patients with decreased baseline SVI, there was no change following SVR. The significant linear relationship between the EDVI and SVI should therefore be considered a surrogate marker of improvement in LV function following SVR (Fig. 9.4a, b).

The improvements in systolic function following SVR have been documented along with improvements in the ventriculoarterial coupling. However, These studies have demonstrated significant perturbations in diastolic function. This could reflect on the surgical technique of geometric restoration. Improvements in ventricular shape have been documented following the use of elliptical intraventricular patches which have a significant bearing on the clinical course and mortality. The adage that optimal function follows optimal form has been emphasized often. The restoration of a physiological ventricular form by the technique of EVLPP has been documented. The existence of the Frank–Starling law in the surgically restored heart by the EVLPP technique has also been well documented. Hemodynamic studies following surgical ventricular restoration techniques which emphasize left ventricular shape restoration rather than only volume reduction need documentation.

References

1. Shapira OM, Davidoff R, Hilkert RJ, Aldea GS, Fitzgerald CA, Shemin RA. Repair of left ventricular aneurysm: long term results of linear repair versus endoaneurysmorraphy. Ann Thorac Surg. 1997;63:701–5.
2. Pocar M, Di Mauro A, Massolunghe D, Monneta A, Megali A, Alsheirei TA, Bregasi A, Matteoli R, Donatelli F. Predictors of adverse events after surgical ventricular restoration for advanced ischemic cardiomyopathy. Eur J Cardiothorac Surg. 2010;37:1093–100.
3. Tiscler MD, Niggel J, Borowski DT, Le Winter MM. Relation between left ventricular shape and exercise capacity in patients with left ventricular dysfunction. J Am Coll Cardiol. 1993;22:751–7.
4. Sabbah HN, Konno T, Stein PD, Mancini GB, Goldstein S. Left ventricular shape changes during the course of evolving heart failure. Am J Physiol. 1992;263(1):H266–70.
5. Tulner SAF, Steendjik P, Klautz RJM, Bax JJ, Shalij MJ, Wall EVD. SVR in patients with ischemic dilated cardiomyopathy: evaluation of systolic and diastolic ventricular function, wall stress, dyssynchrony and mechanical efficiency by pressure–volume loops. J Thorac Cardiovasc Surg. 2006;132:610–20.
6. Kawachi K, Kitamura S, Kawata T, Morita R, Nishii T, Seki T, Taniguchi S, Inoue K. Hemodynamic assessment during exercise after left ventricular aneurysmectomy. J Thorac Cardiovasc Surg. 1994;107:178–83.
7. Tanoue Y, Ando H, Fukumura F, Umesue M, Uchida T, Taniguchi K, Tanaka J. Ventricular energetics in endoventricular circular patch plasty for dyskinetic anterior left ventricular aneurysm. Ann Thorac Surg. 2003;75:1205–8.
8. Stephens JD, Dymond DS, Stone DL, Rees GM, Spurrell RAJ. Left ventricular aneurysm and congestive heart failure: value of exercise stress and isosorbide dinitrate in predicting hemodynamic results of aneurysmectomy. Am J Cardiol. 1980;45:932–9.
9. Artrip JH, Oz MC, Burkhoff D. Left ventricular volume reduction surgery for heart failure: a physiologic perspective. J Thorac Cardiovasc Surg. 2001;122:775–82.
10. Suga H, Sagawa K. Instantaneous pressure-volume relationships and their ratio in the excised, supported canine left ventricle. Circ Res. 1974;35:117–26.
11. Burkhoff D, et al. Surgical ventricular remodeling: a balancing act on systolic and diastolic properties. J Thorac Cardiovasc Surg. 2006;132:459–63.
12. ten Brinke EA, Klautz RJ, Tulner SA, Verwey HF, Bax JJ, Schalij MJ, van der Wall EE, Versteegh MI, Dion RA, Steendijk P. Long-term effects of surgical ventricular restoration with additional restrictive mitral annuloplasty and/or coronary artery bypass grafting on left ventricular function: six-month follow-up by pressure–volume loops. J Thorac Cardiovasc Surg. 2010;140:1338–44.
13. Menicanti L, Di Donato M. The Dor procedure: what has changed after fifteen years of clinical practice? J Thorac Cardiovasc Surg. 2002;124:886.
14. Di Donato M, Sabatier M, Dor V, Gensini GF, Toso A, Maioli M, Stanley AWH, Athanasuleas C, Buckberg G. Effects of the Dor procedure on left ventricular dimension and shape and geometric correlates of mitral regurgitation one year after surgery. J Thorac Cardiovasc Surg. 2001;121:91–6.
15. Castelvecchio S, Menicanti L, Ranucci M, Di Donato M. Impact of surgical ventricular restoration on diastolic function: implications of shape and residual ventricular size. Ann Thorac Surg. 2008;86:1849–54.
16. Fantini F, Barletta G, Toso A, Baroni M, Di Donato M, Sabatier M, Dor V. Effects of reconstructive surgery for left ventricular anterior aneurysm on ventriculoarterial coupling. Heart. 1999;81:171–6.
17. Di Donato MM, Toso A, Dor V, Sabatier M, Barletta G, Menicanti L, Fantini F, and the RESTORE group. Surgical ventricular restoration improves mechanical intraventricular dyssynchrony in ischemic cardiomyopathy. Circulation. 2004;109:2536–43.

18. Biederman RWW, Doyle M. The contribution of CMR to patients undergoing the surgical ventricular restoration (SVR) procedure; one center's experience over five years. Open Magn Reson. 2009;2:33–45.
19. Biederman R, Doyle M, Young A. Global and regional mechanics together with reverse remodeling after LV reconstruction surgery: a one year 3-D MRI analysis. J Cardiovasc Magn Reson. 2002;4:142–3.
20. Adhyapak SM, Parachuri VR. Lessons from a mathematical hypothesis – modification of the endoventricular circular patch plasty. Eur J Cardiothorac Surg. 2011;39:945–51.
21. Jacob R, Dierberger B, Gulch RW, Kissling G. Geometric and muscle physiologic factors of the Frank–Starling mechanism. Basic Res Cardiol. 1993;88:86–91.
22. Jacob R, Gulch RW. The functional significance of ventricular geometry for the transition from hypertrophy to cardiac failure. Does a critical degree of structural dilatation exist? Basic Res Cardiol. 1998;93:423–9.
23. Holubarsch C, Ruf T, Goldstein DJ, Ashton RC, Nickl W, Pieske B, Pioch K, Ludemann J, Weissner S, Hasenfuss G, Poseval H, Just H, Burkhoff D. Existence of the Frank–Starling mechanism in the failing human heart. Circulation. 1996;94:683–9.
24. Mangano DT, Van Dyke DC, Ellis RJ. The effect of increasing pre load on ventricular output and ejection in man. Limitations of the Frank–Starling mechanism. Circulation. 1980;62:535–41.
25. Adhyapak SM, Parachuri VR. Impact of surgical ventricular restoration on stroke volume: surgical fine tuning the relationship between end diastolic volume and stroke volume. J Thorac Cardiovasc Surg. 2011;141(6):1552–3.
26. Renlund DG, Gerstenblith G, Fleg JL, Becker LC, Lakatta EG. Interaction between end diastolic and end systolic volumes in normal humans. Am J Physiol Heart Circ Physiol. 1990;258:H473–81.

10 Recent Controversies: To STICH or Not to STICH?

Introduction

In the light of increasing use of surgical ventricular restoration in patients with advanced heart failure due to large transmural myocardial infarctions and left ventricular aneurysms, who are not eligible for cardiac transplantation, the need for guidelines to direct appropriate standardized therapy was felt. Extensive registry data did document improvements in quality of life with significant decreases in mortality. The surgical procedure underwent an evolutionary change with an expanding surgeon's learning curve from the 1950s to now, documenting nearly 60 years of evolution. The technique of geometric repair was found to be superior to linear plication and excision of the aneurysm in various studies. However, meta-analysis reported favorable results following geometric repair in terms of increased ejection fraction and decreased mortality. But these analyses were plagued by the bias of different time frames of performance of the two surgical techniques, with linear repair being performed earlier and geometric repair later. Hence, these results were confounded by the surgeons' learning curve. There was no randomized study involving surgical ventricular restoration, which was direly needed for guideline formation. In these patients with large left ventricular aneurysms and heart failure, it was necessary to know that if viable, ischemic myocardium was addressed by surgical revascularization and pharmacological therapy alone, there would be resultant decrease in left ventricular dimensions and improvements in function. The issue of whether these patients would require surgical ventricular restoration in addition needed to be addressed.

Need for a Randomized Study Comparing Surgical Ventricular Restoration and Revascularization Alone for Patients with Postinfarction Left Ventricular Dilatation

It has been well established that the ejection fraction does not prognosticate as robustly as the end systolic volume index after an acute myocardial infarction [1]. The degree of left ventricular dilatation predicts mortality and morbidity in ischemic heart disease irrespective of the EF. The presence of stunned or hibernating myocardium following an acute myocardial infarction represents viability which can be restored following revascularization. With the advent of early revascularization, the physical properties of the aneurismal tissues have undergone several changes from fibrous dyskinesis to akinesis which is characterized by islands of viable myocardium within the aneurysm. The border zone also contains viable ischemic tissue which benefits from revascularization. Therefore, to address the issue of whether revascularization alone will benefit those patients with left ventricular aneurysms, leading to reverse remodeling, or there was need for additional ventricular restoration by surgery, a randomized trial was conducted comparing revascularization alone in one arm and revascularization and surgical ventricular restoration

V R. Parachuri, S.M. Adhyapak, *Ventricular Geometry in Post-Myocardial Infarction Aneurysms*,
DOI 10.1007/978-1-4471-2861-8_10,

(SVR) in the other arm. This constituted the hypothesis 2 of the STICH trial [2].

They concluded that surgical ventricular restoration provided no added clinical benefit above revascularization alone. This study may potentially alter treatment of congestive heart failure (CHF) after ischemic dilated cardiomyopathy following myocardial infarction because the authors concluded that adding surgical ventricular reconstruction to reduce ventricular volume to coronary artery bypass grafting (CABG) does not improve symptoms or exercise tolerance and fails to lower death rate or cardiac rehospitalization.

Several registry data have proven differently. Dor [3] showed that the SVR procedure excludes the underlying culprit scar that causes stretch of compensating remote muscle, identified similar regional noncontraction from either aneurysm or akinetic segments that received thrombolysis or angioplasty, and demonstrated that rebuilding left ventricular (LV) size and shape toward normal improves cardiac efficiency by restoring remote muscle function. The keynote finding of similarly absent function in aneurysm without reperfusion (in which the thinned scar collapses during venting) and akinesia after reperfusion (in which the thick myocardium with inner shell scar is covered by normal anterior myocardium that does not collapse during venting) introduced a "new SVR target" with similar beneficial results. This database demonstrates favorable survival compared with CHF natural history studies [4] and a CABG patient cohort whose abnormal ejection fraction and class III/IV New York Heart Association classification matched the RESTORE (Reconstructive Endoventricular Surgery, returning Torsion Original Radius Elliptical Shape) group registry cohort [5, 6] in National Heart, Lung, and Blood Institute STICH grant application and the worldwide SVR registry.

The STICH Trial Components and Study Design

1. The exclusion of the culprit scar with nonviable regions confirmed by nuclear scans to avoid confusion of hibernation within viable muscle.
2. The participating cardiologists had to measure volume in trial entry patients with ejection fractions of less than 35%, since differing volumes may have a similar ejection fraction.
3. The surgeons had to incise the normal epicardium over underlying thick-walled scar and reduce volume 30% below baseline levels. This amount of volume reduction was selected because approximately 40% volume reduction was needed for clinical improvement in prior SVR reports of more than 5,000 patients.
4. STICH measured volume in only 161 of 490 SVR patients. No evaluation could be made in 66% of SVR patients whose volume was not measured.
5. CHF severity reached grade III/IV (New York Heart Association) in only 49% of patients in the STICH cohort versus approximately 67% in SVR registry reports.
6. The LV end systolic volume index (ESVI) should be greater than 60 mL/m^2.
7. The documentation of greater than 35% akinesia from anterior wall necrosis was necessary to show that the culprit scar caused remote muscle dilatation that exceeded the 60 mL/m^2 entry point.
8. Revised amendment of "documented LV anterior wall dysfunction" was done if necrosis and volume measurements were absent. This was because 13% of patients had not had a myocardial infarction. These primary goal amendments introduced wall motion disorders that may occur without necrosis after acute ischemia or hibernation or may follow scar. Ischemic muscle without scar may recover after CABG, but this cannot happen if gadolinium magnetic resonance studies show that greater than 50% of muscle is scarred.

SVR has never been recommended in ventricles without scar, and applying SVR in hibernating myocardium was not reported by Dor in more than 1,000 patients or the 1,198 RESTORE patient cohort in which all patients displayed electrocardiographic and imaging evidence of large akinetic or dyskinetic scar with greater than 60 mL/m^2 ESVI measurements. Echocardiography was used to measure LV volume in the *STICH* report but was evaluated in only 38% of STICH patients (212/490 CABG patients and 161/490 CABG and SVR patients).

LV volume was reduced by 19% in SVR patients to reach a volume end point that reflected an inadequate repair as determined by the Surgery Therapy Committee, whose "acceptable STICH procedure" guideline required a 30% ESVI decrease at 4-month CMR measurement. Consequently, the STICH SVR procedure may have reflected a small LV plication or limited intracavitary reconstruction.

STICH Trial Flaws

The credibility of the STICH trial is questioned by its various flaws:

1. All patients needed to have akinesia, yet only 50% displayed this finding.
2. Akinesia developed from regional necrosis of 35% of muscle, yet the report fails to document this scar finding.
3. CMR quantification of ventricular volume is needed in all patients before and after SVR. Instead, 19% underwent an invalid echocardiographic measurement despite pretrial contact showing CMR measurement capacity in all initial 50 trial centers.
4. All patients required CMR volume measurement for trial entry, yet only 38% (CABG and CABG plus SVR) had any form of volume measurement.
5. SVR is indicated only if ESVI is beyond 60 mL/m^2, yet volume measurements for SVR or CABG without SVR candidates were not reported.
6. A 30% reduction of ESVI at 4 months by CMR study is required for acceptable SVR procedure, but ESVI was lowered only 19% in the 33% of patients which demonstrated an inadequate end point.
7. The original trial included 50 centers, averaging approximately 10 cases per center. Actually, 96 centers were used, averaging approximately 5 procedures per center, so that Surgical Therapy Committee outcome validation during accreditation becomes a vital earmark before trial enrollment. Its initial meeting outlined ten cases per center and five per surgeon, demonstrating the required 30% volume reduction. Instead, no specification is shown that pretrial ESVI reduction fulfilled trial eligibility criteria.

The hallmark of technical competence after any surgical procedure requires reaching goals that comply with yardsticks of procedural success. For SVR, favorable clinical results followed approximately 40% volume reduction below control levels in more than 1,500 cases in 12 worldwide centers. In contrast, STICH reduced ventricular volume 19% in 161 patients, and 96 centers were required to achieve this end point. No volume studies occurred in 66% of patients, and an invalid echo-based monitoring method was used in the others. These limitations did not prevent STICH end point interpretation that SVR should be abandoned because CABG achieved similar results. What these results do not consider is how they relate to evaluation of unapproved volume outcomes in only 33% of patients or how experience influences end point validity.

These potentially inaccurate conclusions of volume reduction could be documented by comparing STICH to the 1976 Veterans Administration Hospital CABG study [7] of ischemic coronary artery disease revascularization versus medical therapy. The 300 surgically treated patients in 12 centers had 6% mortality (range 3–12%) and closed conduits related to individual center experience. This contrasts with 1% mortality and superb graft patency in a 1978 report of 1,000 patients from the Cleveland Clinic [8] to demonstrate how experience-based observations influence subsequent management. STICH trial inexperience potential may relate to the learning curve of adequately reducing ventricular volume while doing a new procedure when only about five cases per center are performed.

The technique of SVR may also affect the outcomes of surgery, just as the experience of the operator does. As already discussed in the previous chapters, the technique of endoventricular circular patch plasty (EVCPP) results in a smaller ventricle which continues to be more spherical than the normal physiological ellipsoid.

Misguided results may camouflage proper outcome analysis and negatively influence future correct treatment in the same way that coronary revascularization can be considered unsuccessful when only internal thoracic artery grafting is done without addressing a stenotic right coronary artery or concluding that antihypertensive drugs are ineffective in studies that used inadequate medication dosages.

We believe that differences between STICH outcomes and worldwide SVR data displaying greater volume reduction indicate that the wrong operation, using the wrong volume measurement monitors, was done on the wrong patients and resulted in the wrong conclusions. This outcome deprives cardiologists of understanding the potential role of volume reduction to treat CHF from ischemic dilated cardiomyopathy and demonstrates that the *goals* of evidence-based medicine were not achieved.

The STICH end points do not relate to the SVR procedure that requires properly measuring necrosis and accurate ventricular volume before reducing volume more than 30% below preoperative levels.

This trial may adversely affect cardiac surgery evolution and nontransplant heart failure surgery by limiting development of SVR, a unifying geometric treatment of dilated cardiomyopathy from ischemic and nonischemic causes. The procedure of SVR may link with LV assist devices to introduce a "bridge to restoration" approach and ultimately may create a surgical scaffold that unites a macroscopic approach with cell therapy in the future. The ultimate blow is to scientific integrity because measuring volume rather than ejection fraction as the natural surrogate for development of adverse clinical findings in dilated hearts becomes impaired by STICH findings.

Despite CABG, LV volumes typically increase with a commensurate increase in the persistence of heart failure and an earlier than predicted mortality. Further debate over whether resting myocardial blood flow is abnormal in "hibernating" myocardium or whether "hibernation" represents repetitive "stunning" is the topic of much current discussion in the scientific community [9].

What has become clear is that the myocardium in ischemic cardiomyopathy is made up of a combination of scarred, hibernating, and stunned myocardium. Within a given region of scar, there may exist patches or islands of viable myocardium. Once this is understood, it becomes clear why cardiac CMR is an ideal choice for the non-invasive assessment of myocardial viability.

The Unanswered Questions

1. Incorrect volume measurements were used, along with incomplete assessment of ventricular volumes.
2. Does CABG treatment lead to improved function in scarred muscle? CABG is used in the non-SVR group that does not exclude the scarred segment.
3. The viability measurements showing 35% regional necrosis in all included patients are absent.
4. There was no confirmed validation of center–surgeon eligibility greater than 30% volume reduction to comply with Surgical Therapy Committee guidelines.
5. The grey zone of areas of ischemia (with or without hibernation) and postmyocardial infarction anterior scar were not clearly differentiated.
6. With all these inaccuracies and fallacies, the procedure of SVR cannot be invalidated as against the extensive evidence from the SVR patient registry database.

The suggestions by Buckberg and Athanasuleas [10] are:

The target goal must (1) exclude all patients with invalid echocardiographic volume measurements, (2) include only patients in whom regional nonviability of greater than 35% akinesia is documented by nuclear medicine scans, (3) quantify all patients with greater than 30% volume reduction by CMR study, and (4) report only patients with "acceptable" volume reduction by CMR at 4 months. The STICH trial must address each of these questions because misguided STICH conclusions contradict the role of augmented ventricular volume as the surrogate for the natural history of increasing morbidity and mortality in dilated hearts. Without this action, the STICH trial conclusions simply show that statisticians can defy nature from a flawed database.

References

1. White HD, Norris RM, Brown MA, Brandt PW, Whitlock RM, Wild CJ. Left ventricular end-systolic volume as the major determinant of survival after recovery from myocardial infarction. Circulation. 1987;76:44–51.
2. Jones RH, Velazquez EJ, Michler RE, Sopko G, Oh JK, O'Connor CM, et al. Coronary bypass surgery with or without surgical ventricular reconstruction. N Engl J Med. 2009;360:1705–17.
3. Dor V. Left ventricular reconstruction: the aim and the reality after twenty years. J Thorac Cardiovasc Surg. 2004;128:17–20.
4. Levy D, Kenchaiah S, Larson MG, Benjamin EJ, Kupka MJ, Ho KK, et al. Long-term trends in the incidence of and survival with heart failure. N Engl J Med. 2002;347:1397–402.
5. Athanasuleas CL, Buckberg GD, Stanley AW, Siler W, Dor V, Di Donato M, for the RESTORE group, et al. Surgical ventricular restoration in the treatment of congestive heart failure due to post-infarction ventricular dilation. J Am Coll Cardiol. 2004;44:1439–45.
6. Shah PJ, Hare DL, Raman JS, Gordon I, Chan RK, Horowitz JD, et al. Survival after myocardial revascularization for ischemic cardiomyopathy: a prospective ten-year follow-up study. J Thorac Cardiovasc Surg. 2003;126:1320–7.
7. Takaro T, Hultgren HN, Lipton MJ, Detre KM. The VA cooperative randomized study of surgery for coronary arterial occlusive disease II. Subgroup with significant left main lesions. Circulation. 1976;54:III107–17.
8. Sheldon WC, Loop FD, Proudfit WL. A critique of the VA cooperative study. Cleve Clin Q. 1978;45:225–30.
9. Kloner RA, Bolli R, Marban E, et al. Medical and cellular implications of stunning, hibernation, and preconditioning: an NHLBI Workshop. Circulation. 1998;97:1848–67.
10. Buckberg GD, Athanasuleas CL. The STICH trial: misguided conclusions. J Thorac Cardiovasc Surg. 2009;138:1060–4.

Role of Electrophysiological Testing, Intracardiac Defibrillator Implantation, and Concomitant Surgical Procedures in Patients with Left Ventricular Aneurysms Presenting with Ventricular Tachycardia

11

V Rao Parachuri, Srilakshmi M. Adhyapak, and A.G. Ravi Kishore

Introduction

Although the occurrence of sudden cardiac death has decreased substantially after surgical ventricular restoration, its persistence in some patients is a cause of immense concern. These patients constitute a different subset from the patients enrolled in the MADIT trials. The patients eligible for the MADIT trial with subsequent ICD implantation were selected solely on the basis of left ventricular ejection fraction. These patients did not have distinct left ventricular aneurysms and areas of contractile myocardium.

The associated procedure of cryoablation and endocardiectomy in addition to surgical ventricular restoration has been tried with commendable success in patients with left ventricular aneurysms. However, the patient selection for this procedure continues to be based on the clinical judgment of the treating physician and surgeon. In the scenario of overt tachyarrhythmias, there is no doubt of adding cryoablation. But, in the situation where the clinical presentation does not include tachyarrhythmias, the indications for electrophysiological testing (EP testing) are not very clear and are based on the clinical judgment of the treating physician. This gray zone, and the scenario of postoperative EP testing, calls for formulation of guidelines to treat this difficult subset of patients. Here, we discuss the various reasons for occurrence of ventricular tachyarrhythmias in this patient population and the treatment modalities which have been used previously and those in vogue now for the same, highlighting our approach.

V R. Parachuri, FRCS (CTh) (✉)
Heart Lung Transplantation Program,
Narayana Hrudayalaya Institute of Medical Sciences,
258/A, Bommaasandra Industrial Area, Anekal Taluk,
Bangalore Karnataka 560099, India
e-mail: hellorao@gmail.com

S.M. Adhyapak, DNB
Department of Cardiology,
St. John's Medical College Hospital,
Bangalore, Karnataka 560034, India
e-mail: srili2881967@yahoo.com

A.G.R. Kishore, DM
Department of Electrophysiology and arrhythmias,
Narayana Hrudayalaya Institute of Medical Sciences,
258/A, Bommasandra Industrial Area, Anekal Taluk,
Bangalore, Karnataka 560099, India
e-mail: ravikishoreag@yahoo.co.in

V R. Parachuri, S.M. Adhyapak, *Ventricular Geometry in Post-Myocardial Infarction Aneurysms*,
DOI 10.1007/978-1-4471-2861-8_11,

Mechanisms of Ventricular Tachyarrhythmias in Postinfarct Left Ventricular Aneurysms

Mechanism of Reentry

The mechanism of ventricular tachyarrhythmias in ischemic cardiomyopathy is mostly due to the reentry phenomenon, the focus of which is at the border zone of infarcted and uninfarcted myocardium. The ability to reproducibly initiate an arrhythmia by programmed ventricular stimulation (PVS) on EP testing is considered a characteristic of reentrant arrhythmia and is the mechanism of sustained uniform VT associated with coronary artery disease [1]. Both nonsustained and sustained polymorphic arrhythmias, including ventricular fibrillation, can be induced even in persons without cardiac disease. However, in a person with cardiac disease or even a history of cardiac arrest, induction of polymorphic VT can have a clinical significance because a cardiac arrest may be initiated by a polymorphic VT. More importantly, the induction of a sustained uniform tachycardia only occurs in patients with spontaneous VT or cardiac arrest or in the presence of a substrate known to be arrhythmogenic such as a left ventricular aneurysm or recent myocardial infarction [2]. The possibility of inducing VT increases with decreasing LV function, and patients with depressed LV function and inducible sustained VT have a higher risk of spontaneous VT than those who do not have inducible VT [3, 4].

Mechanoelectrical Mechanism of Arrhythmia Genesis

Another mechanism has been proposed which is related to the amount ventricular stretch. This has been identified as a mechanoelectrical component which generates and propagates ventricular tachyarrhythmias. The degree of ventricular stretch in patients with ventricular dilatation has been implicated in this phenomenon. The basis for this has been studied by Lab and coworkers by in vitro studies [5]. This has been interpreted as Lab's Occam's razor hypothesis.

The English theologian and philosopher William of Occam (1280–1349) stated "Entia non sunt multiplicanda praeter necessitatum." This is recognized as Occam's razor. Roughly interpreted, it proposes that it is better to have one hypothesis to explain five observations than five hypotheses to explain each one. The cardiovascular clinical parameters used for predicting sudden arrhythmic death ranging through indices of neurohormonal status (i.e., heart rate variability) to indices of electrophysiological substrate (i.e., late potentials, QT dispersion, alternans) are influenced by and associated with mechanical disturbances in the heart. The cardiac action potential widens with ventricular dilatation. With the onset of heart failure, an increase in intracellular calcium can trigger ventricular ectopics. These can be recognized as ventricular afterdepolarizations on the surface ECG. Patients with more extensive cardiac remodeling are more prone to ventricular tachyarrhythmias and sudden death. This occurs due to the marked inhomogeneity of impulse propagation through normally contracting myocardium and areas of marked inhomogenous contractions.

The clinical background for the role of LV dilation as a basic factor stems from (1) the capacity of early reperfusion after myocardial infarction to reduce both extent of dilation during remodeling (by shrinking the dyskinetic heart to a smaller akinetic chamber) and early arrhythmia development, (2) the positive correlation of increasing evidence for ventricular arrhythmia as LVESVI increases [6], (3) failure of antiremodeling drugs (beta blocker and ACE inhibitors) to limit arrhythmias in stretched hearts that do not alter dilation [6], or (4) antiarrhythmic drugs to prevent progression of arrhythmia formation [6]. The prognostic importance of ventricular arrhythmias is underlined by the resultant extensive use of ICD to reduce this cause of 50% mortality, a treatment that directly deals with this electrical complication in dilated hearts. In contrast, the capacity of volume reduction and shape alteration to markedly offset this complication may provide a clinical series that supports Lab's Occam's razor principle suggesting that mechanoelectric events create a central hypothesis for ventricular arrhythmias in remodeled hearts [5].

Global mechanoelectric ventricular stretch may be the vital clinical factor, since a similar lethal complication causes 50% of deaths following spherical volume increment in valvular heart disease patients who do not have the underlying fibrosis that exists following myocardial infarction [7–9].

Surgical Treatment Modalities for Ventricular Tachyarrhythmias in the Pre-ICD Era

Left ventricular aneurysm is a serious complication of acute myocardial infarction associated with congestive heart failure and ventricular tachycardia (VT). Ventricular arrhythmias after myocardial infarctions are associated with high mortality and risk for sudden cardiac death [3, 4]. Left ventricular aneurysm represents an independent predictor of late sudden cardiac death [10].

Mortality in patients with heart failure after cardiac dilation and impaired ejection fraction is due to progressive heart failure in about 50% of patients and by sudden death in the other 50% of patients [11]. Recent studies indicate that monomorphic premature ventricular contractions originating from the scar border zone in ischemic cardiomyopathy can be triggers for ventricular fibrillation [12]. Early surgical attempts to treat refractory VT have been associated with high failure rates [13, 14]. Coronary artery bypass graft surgery alone does not eliminate the risk of ventricular arrhythmias in ischemic heart disease, especially not in the presence of poor LV function [15, 16].

To address this devastating arrhythmic complication, in the pre-implantable cardioverter-defibrillator (ICD) era, Dor and associates presented an addition to the original operation [17] which was map-guided endocardial resection, in patients with VT, with a success rate of greater than >90% in curing VT [18]. Other centers have reported similar results using a map-guided approach and the Dor procedure [19]. The concomitant surgical techniques for ventricular tachyarrhythmias, in this era, included map- or non-map-guided endocardial resection with or without LV aneurysmectomy, encircling cryoablation at the border zone, and revascularization.

However, the frequency of recurrence, complexity of mapped guided interventions, and high rates of spontaneous and inducible ventricular tachycardia (VT) in postinfarction patients identified the persistence of risk of sudden cardiac death. In addition, there was a high incidence of sudden death (37% of 19 deaths during median follow-up of 3.7 years) late after anterior SVR when concomitant antiarrhythmic surgery was not performed [20].

MADIT Trial in Ischemic Cardiomyopathy

This arrhythmic component in ischemic cardiomyopathy with heart failure was assessed in the multicenter automatic defibrillator implantation trial (MADIT II), where implantable cardioverter-defibrillator (ICD) therapy saved sudden death in high-risk coronary patients with advanced left ventricular dysfunction [45]. This electrical approach did not adequately address nonsudden death from progression of heart failure. In this trial, the criterion for ICD implantation consisted of evidence of prior transmural infarction and left ventricular ejection fraction ≤30%. This trial did not target patients with large and discrete left ventricular aneurysms and patients with ischemic cardiomyopathy with LVEF >30%.

Surgical Ventricular Restoration and Ventricular Tachyarrhythmias

The initiation of ventricular size reduction to treat ventricular arrhythmias stemmed from Dor's observation that reduced ventricular arrhythmias were associated with his efforts to improve pump function after surgical correction of akinetic or dyskinetic scar after myocardial infarction. This could have been the result of mechanical resynchronization with exclusion of large scarred areas of myocardium.

Subsequently, patients with spontaneous and or inducible arrhythmias underwent subtotal endocardial resection and encircling cryoablation at the border of the lesion. Consequently, patients without spontaneous or inducible ventricular tachycardia underwent only surgical ventricular restoration.

When the patients who had concomitant arrhythmia surgery for preoperative spontaneous or inducible VT were subjected to EP studies postoperatively, only 8% of the patients that were 100% inducible before surgery were inducible postoperatively.

Di Donato and coworkers demonstrated that in patients with clinical arrhythmias at baseline, the incidence of postoperative induction was only 16%, yet some noninducible patients developed new postoperative inducible ventricular tachycardia [11].

Thus, the presence of postoperative arrhythmias in patients who were noninducible preoperatively questions the role of EP studies as a risk stratifier for concomitant arrhythmia surgery. But, the induction of a sustained uniform tachycardia only occurs in patients with spontaneous VT or cardiac arrest or in the presence of a substrate known to be arrhythmogenic such as a left ventricular aneurysm or recent myocardial infarction [2]. The possibility of inducing VT increases with decreasing LV function, and patients with depressed LV function and inducible sustained VT have a higher risk of spontaneous VT than those who do not have inducible VT [3, 4]. This fact also cannot be ignored, as well as the persistent incidence of late sudden death after SVR when concomitant arrhythmia surgery was not performed which has been mentioned above.

This constitutes the gray zone of testing for inducibility in patients without spontaneous VT.

Role of Electrophysiology in Patients with Left Ventricular Aneurysms

EP testing prior to surgery is performed solely at the discretion of the treating physician, as there are no guideline recommendations for the same in this subset of patients. The EP study is performed using programmed ventricular stimulation. The stimulation protocols consist of programmed ventricular stimulation with either (1) up to three ventricular extrastimuli, after eight-beat paced drive cycles at up to two paced cycle lengths at two right ventricular endocardial sites, or (2) four extrastimuli at three paced cycle lengths at two right ventricular sites. Burst pacing, short-long-short coupling intervals, or both can also be performed. The specific stimulation protocol is at the discretion of the physician.

A positive study is defined as inducible sustained ventricular tachyarrhythmias (monomorphic or polymorphic) lasting more than 30 s or associated with syncope, hemodynamic compromise, or the necessity for intervention for termination. A negative EP study is defined as noninducibility of sustained ventricular tachyarrhythmias. The decision to implant an ICD is made on the basis of late (>48 h) documented life-threatening ventricular arrhythmias after SVR (secondary prevention of sudden cardiac death) or for a positive EP study (primary prevention).

Although programmed ventricular stimulation is a diagnostic tool to assess efficacy of treatment and stratify the risk of sudden death, there exist significant concerns about its utility as a risk stratifier [21, 22] Currently, ICD implantation is employed in class II–III patients with ischemic cardiomyopathy and low ejection fraction, and spontaneous or PVS inducible arrhythmias, but class IV CHF patients are excluded.

Without surgical ventricular restoration (SVR), sudden death prevention by ICD implantation is superior to mapping-guided pharmacological treatment. However, ventricular tachyarrhythmias associated with the SVR procedure showed that postoperative risk of sudden death from ventricular arrhythmias was similar in patients with and without spontaneous and inducible ventricular tachycardia. Endocardiectomy and cryoablation were used whenever there is spontaneous arrhythmia or if preoperative PVS showed inducible ventricular arrhythmias.

In Di Donato's series [11], only one ICD was needed, and the use of amiodarone following positive postoperative PVS yielded high survival and a low rate of sudden death. This benefit of amiodarone may relate to how volume and shape reduction during SVR differs from nonsurgical approaches that are characterized by progressive volume increase during ongoing remodeling [6].

Apart from the diagnostic usefulness of EP studies, PVS was not a useful risk stratifier, since the postoperative SVR findings showed limited sudden deaths following inducible tachycardia. Sudden death was a more common cause of mortality (16%) in patients with noninducible arrhythmias than in patients with inducible VT and subsequent concomitant arrhythmic surgery (8%).

These results are similar to the follow-up MADIT II trial data findings, where patients who were not inducible at EPS had greater ventricular fibrillation-related use of ICD therapy than those who were inducible.

The MADIT II trial reports an incidence of sudden cardiac death in 61% of conventional group against 35% in the defibrillator group, whereas the SVR data summary showed SVR patients dying of sudden death (18.7% of all deaths) when volume reduction was used to alter the ventricular stretch and shape factors. The sudden cardiac death rate in the MADIT ICD group was 3.8% and 10% in the conventional group. In contrast, the SVR sudden cardiac death rate was 2.5% and thereby lower than that in both MADIT II groups.

Sudden Cardiac Death and Nonsudden Cardiac Death due to Worsening Heart Failure in the MADIT II Patients

In the MADIT II, the nonsudden cardiac deaths in the ICD group was significantly higher than deaths in the conventional group (55% vs. 26%), especially during the first year. Furthermore, the adverse cardiac event of congestive heart failure during the week preceding cardiac death was 43% in the ICD group versus 16% in the conventional-treated group. This suggests that non-cardiac death may be caused by progressive heart failure in these patients, and sudden death accounts for about 50% of deaths in this population, and ICD limited only the arrhythmia component. However, ICD did not sufficiently address the underlying progressive remodeling, a structural event that defines the positive correlation between progressive stretch and ventricular arrhythmia development [6].

Mechanoelectrical Component Responsible for Nonsudden Cardiac Death due to Worsening Heart Failure in Patients with Left Ventricular Aneurysms

The mechanoelectric event of chamber stretching may be a critical mechanistic factor that causes this lethal rhythm complication. This dilation and shape finding is not changed by ICD utilization, so that the electrical treatment mode only addresses the arrhythmic symptom of this terminal electrical event.

The MADIT data cannot be compared with SVR, but sudden cardiac death in this restoration study population is much lower than after ICD, and Kaplan–Meier estimates for cardiac death do not show differences between SVR patients with and without preoperative ventricular arrhythmias. Consequently, Di Donato et al. [11] concluded that ICD is not needed when a surgical rebuilding approach is undertaken. Unfortunately, the combination of cryoablation, endocardiectomy, CABG, and mitral repair does not allow clear distinction of how volume reduction and shape alteration specifically contributed to reduced arrhythmias.

Reduction of LV cavity size with septal and scar exclusion would prevent functioning of the reentry circuit [23], and the adequate endocardium resection and large encircling cryoablation during aneurysmectomy would provide a higher electrical success rate [24, 25]. This concept needs further testing, since overall mortality was comparably low in a recent patient cohort from the RESTORE group [26] that did not undergo PVS evaluation.

In contrast, the late deaths reported by Athanasuleas were more common in dilated hearts and presumably arrhythmia-related deaths [26].

This data analysis suggests a close relationship between ventricular volume and arrhythmia development, since spontaneous arrhythmias were greatest in the most dilated hearts (LVESVI>120 mL/m^2), inducible arrhythmias more frequent after lesser dilation (LVESVI between 100 and 120 mL/m^2), and absent in smaller (LVESVI<100 mL/m^2) hearts.

These observations stimulate rethinking in the possible mechanisms of ventricular tachyarrhythmias in these patients. They support Lab's Occam's razor principle analysis of the interaction of volume and ventricular stretch as a potential additional mechanism of arrhythmia development in the dilated failing heart. These clinical correlates have a firm experimental base, since addressing volume alone changed arrhythmic generation and accelerated fibrillation thresholds in stretched left and right ventricles in both acute and chronic laboratory studies [5].

Stretch events may be central in the spectrum of contributory factors in potential lethal ventricular arrhythmias in remodeled ventricles.

SVR creates a mechanical intraventricular resynchronization in patients with ischemic cardiomyopathy and with no preoperative electrical conduction delay [27]. It has also been shown in patients with ischemic cardiomyopathy that cardiac resynchronization therapy reduces both inducibility of VT [28] and frequency of VT episodes [29, 30]. Thus, it seems that intraventricular resynchronization, either by SVR or biventricular pacing, reduces ventricular arrhythmias in the dilated heart. The mechanism for this improvement may be related to the beneficial effects on LV synchrony because improved synchrony will not only improve LV hemodynamics but also homogenize regional wall stress and reduce regional prestretch, which is potentially arrhythmogenic [31]. The option of CRT or cardiac resynchronization therapy by means of biventricular pacing cannot be applied to patients with left ventricular aneurysms. As the indications for this therapy mandates the presence of intraventricular conduction delay on the surface electrocardiogram and has been found to be suboptimal in the presence of large areas of left ventricular scar [32].

The occurrence of late sudden deaths following SVR by EVCPP could be explained by late re-remodeling or redilatation of the ventricle [20]. This explanation is plausible as none of these patients had inducible VT preoperatively. But, the limitation of this study has been the lack of postoperative data of left ventricular volumes. If the presence of arrhythmias can be demonstrated in late re-remodeling after EVCPP, this finding would reflect on the surgical technique of SVR while validating the mechanism of Lab's Occam's razor principle in the generation of ventricular tachyarrhythmias in heart failure with dilated ventricles.

Furthermore, clinical work has defined how LV decompression by left ventricular assist devices (LVAD) positively alters electrophysiologic alterations in patients with advanced heart failure [33]. The overall surgical procedure deals with the vessel (CABG), valve (mitral repair when needed), and ventricle (SVR), together with endocardiectomy and cryoablation, so that one single factor cannot be identified to account for the high electrical success rate in these patients. It is rather difficult to isolate the confounding effects of the three different surgical procedures on arrhythmia production.

Inherent Problems with Intracardiac Map-Guided Cryoablation and Endocardiectomy

Mapping studies in patients with anteroapical scarring showed that the anatomic substrate for ventricular arrhythmias was located in the border zone between scar and surrounding normal endocardium on the ventricular septum [26]. Ablation using endocardial excision often combined with cryoablation or creation of homogeneous scar after attachment of a septal patch controlled the arrhythmia [34].

The procedure of large encircling cryoablation without mapping was done because of observations that, especially with quadripolar handheld electrodes, mapping was not successful in all patients after ventriculotomy (mapping success rate of 63%, unpublished data). Moreover, in the majority of patients with anterior MI, the earliest activation or cryotermination site was located within the area of the visible scar tissue. Although large blind endocardiectomy has produced consistently high success rates, the arduous nature of this procedure—particularly when performed on mitral papillary muscle or interventricular septum—compelled the use of large encircling cryoablation. The electrical success rate based on postoperative electrophysiologic studies was 94.5%. Overall electrical success rate was 89.1%. Freedom from ventricular tachycardia was 77% (95% CI 61–94%) at both 5 and 7 years. Freedom from sudden cardiac death was 91% (95% CI 80–100%) at both 5 and 7 years, with overall actuarial survivals at 5 and 7 years of 63% (95% CI 47–80%) and 42% (95% CI 22–63%), respectively. The main cause of late death was congestive heart failure in 62.6% of these patients which reflects on the long-term adverse effects of endocardiectomy [35].

Clinical Data of Concomitant Surgical Procedures Employed in Various SVR Registries for Ventricular Tachyarrhythmias

The RESTORE findings suggest more late arrhythmias in ventricles >80 mL/m^2, since the incidence of rehospitalization was similar when preoperative LVESVI was <80 or >80 mL/m^2. These observations imply that future trials should evaluate the role of adding endocardiectomy and or direct approaches like cryotherapy in patients with >80 mL/m^2 LVESVI who will undergo SVR to treat ventricular dysfunction.

In their initial study on the outcome of SVR, the Reconstructive Endoventricular Original Radius Elliptical Shape to the Left Ventricle group reported arrhythmic deaths in 4 of 8 late deaths, which occurred in 207 patients who survived to discharge from the hospital after SVR [36].

Dor [17, 34] (who routinely used cryoablation and endocardial resection) reported an 8% incidence of inducible ventricular tachycardia after surgery.

In a Japanese study of SVR employed in patients with only akinetic left ventricular scars, 3 (6%) of 47 died from arrhythmic deaths after discharge [37].

Mickleborough [38] reported a very low incidence of ventricular arrhythmias after left ventricular aneurysmectomy and a 79% 5-year survival. With the use of an intraventricular mapping balloon, they demonstrated that the ease of induction of arrhythmias was critically related to mechanical loading conditions of the heart. As the balloon was inflated, ventricular arrhythmias were induced. Therefore, any procedure that restores ventricular volume and size toward normal (such as ventricular reconstruction) is likely to reduce the inducibility or occurrence of ventricular arrhythmias. They performed map-directed surgery with freedom from sudden death of 97% at 5 years and an overall survival of 79%.

They have included in ventricular reconstruction a visually directed endocardial excision with cryoablation at the periphery in 86 patients who had recurrent ventricular tachycardia preoperatively and inducible ventricular tachycardia at electrophysiologic study. Those with inducible or spontaneous tachycardia postoperatively were discharged on a regimen of amiodarone. During follow-up, arrhythmia recurrence was only rarely a problem. Only one patient in the entire series required an ICD, and freedom from sudden death or recurrent ventricular tachycardia was 99% at 1 year and 96% at 5 years. They concluded that a combination of revascularization and ventricular reconstruction appeared to be very effective in preventing arrhythmia recurrence in these patients.

Bechtel et al. [20] reported that the postoperative presence of ventricular tachyarrhythmias necessitating treatment was an independent risk factor for sudden cardiac death. Out of 34 inhospital survivors who experienced ventricular tachyarrhythmias early postoperatively, 26 were alive at follow-up and 8 had died, 3 of whom were sudden.

Frapier and colleagues [39] have reported the results of encircling cryoablation for recurrent ventricular tachycardia.

The procedure was done with the aid of cardioplegic arrest, through left ventriculotomy through the scar, as first described by Guiraudon and associates [40], without mapping. Points of cryolesion were either edge to edge or overlapping and applied 1.5 cm outside the area of the visible scar in all patients. In the septum, where the exact delimitation of the scar is less easy, this distance of 1.5 cm was increased so that a second row could be applied. Care was taken to avoid ablation in the upper part of the septum near its membranous portion, which can cause a His bundle block (which happened twice at the beginning of their experience). Cryoablation was performed with a Frigitronics cryosurgical system CCS 100 with a 15-mm-diameter flat-face curved probe (Cooper Surgical Inc, Shelton, Conn). A mean of 11.4 ± 2.2 cryolesions (range 8–15) was realized at a mean temperature of −61°C (range −50°C to −74°C) for 2 min per point.

Our Experience with Concomitant Linear Cryoablation

At our Institution, we have performed cryoablation on six patients who presented with spontaneous VT [41, 42]. We have not conducted EP testing for inducibility in patients who did not present with spontaneous VT. None of our patients underwent preoperative EP testing for inducibility. Our principle of linear cryoablation was modeled after the technique of radiofrequency ablation for ventricular tachycardia. As ventricular tachycardia in scarred ventricles is predominantly due to macroreentry at the border zone, linear radiofrequency ablation applied longitudinally from the ventricular base (mitral annulus) toward the apex (inferior aspect of the apical scar) successfully breaks the macroreentrant circuit.

Our procedure of cryoablation was performed with a cryosurgical system using a Deluxe AA3 probe equipped with a curved tip (Appasamy Associates, Chennai, India). It was done before securing the linear endoventricular patch within the ventricular cavity, in a linear fashion starting from the posterior mitral annulus to the inferior aspect of the apical scar which was the area of securing the endoventricular patch later, for exclusion of the scarred myocardium. The linear cryoablation was achieved with application of a temperature of −60° for 2 min at each point. We do not advocate the encircling cryoablation in ventricles with extensive scar tissue, as delineation of scar tissue may be difficult. The other technical hindrance is the presence of deep and extensive muscular trabeculae within the left ventricular cavity, where application of encircling cryoablation may be difficult. Several surgeons have felt that encircling cryoablation is cumbersome with the endoventricular patch in situ and may lead to worsening left ventricular dysfunction with increasing mortality from heart failure per se [35]. The procedure of endocardiectomy is also fraught with its attendant complications.

All our patients were subjected to EP studies at 6 weeks to 6 months after surgery, and none demonstrated inducibility of ventricular tachyarrhythmias on PVS. None of our patients demonstrated re-remodeling late after SVR. All patients demonstrated persistent late reverse remodeling, with further decreases in left ventricular end diastolic and end systolic volumes and increases in left ventricular ejection fractions. None of the six patients who underwent linear cryoablation had recurrence of ventricular tachyarrhythmias, inducibility on postoperative EP testing, and there was no mortality among this subset in our cohort.

Clinical Outcomes of EP Testing and ICD Implantation in Patients Undergoing SVR: The Cleveland Experience

James O' Neill [43] and coworkers have studied patients undergoing SVR at the Cleveland Clinic prospectively to determine the role of ICD implantation following SVR. This study was undertaken as there are no clear guidelines regarding the necessity of early ICD implantation in patients undergoing SVR. Patients were divided into three groups: *group 1*, implantable cardioverter-defibrillator present before surgery; *group 2*, implantable cardioverter-defibrillator implanted early after surgery; and *group 3*, no implantable cardioverter-defibrillator implanted.

EP testing was performed on most patients before discharge, at the discretion of the treating physician. The EP study was performed using programmed ventricular stimulation. The stimulation protocols consisted of programmed ventricular stimulation with either (1) up to three ventricular extrastimuli, after eight-beat paced drive cycles at up to two paced cycle lengths at two right ventricular endocardial sites, or (2) four extrastimuli at three paced cycle lengths at two right ventricular sites. Burst pacing, short-long-short coupling intervals, or both were also performed in some patients. The specific stimulation protocol was at the discretion of the physician. A positive study was defined as inducible sustained ventricular tachyarrhythmias (monomorphic or polymorphic) lasting more than 30 s or associated with syncope, hemodynamic compromise, or the necessity for intervention for termination. A negative EP study was defined as noninducibility of sustained ventricular tachyarrhythmias. The decision to implant an ICD was made on the basis of late (>48 h) documented life-threatening ventricular arrhythmias after SVR (secondary prevention of sudden cardiac death) or for a positive EP study (primary prevention).

Their results demonstrated that patients remained at high risk for ventricular tachyarrhythmias following SVR. Among patients who underwent EP studies, 42% tested positive for inducible sustained ventricular arrhythmias. In patients with ICDs, 15% had either sudden cardiac death or appropriate ICD shocks. ICD therapies tended to occur early, within the first 60–90 days. With the strategy of early EP study, ICD implantation, or both, the overall incidence of sudden death was <1%. The effects of EP studies and ICD therapies have not been analyzed in other studies of SVR, including a large observational study (surgical anterior ventricular endocardial restoration) of 439 patients undergoing SVR [26].

Whether EP risk stratification or ICD implantation without EP testing is warranted before discharge after SVR is a matter of extensive debate. In light of MADIT II, the utility of EP studies in patients with coronary disease and ejection fractions <30% has been questioned because the benefit of ICD implantation occurs irrespective of EP testing. In the population presented here, however, negative EP studies were predictive of good 30-day survival. No patient with a negative EP study died within 30 days (two died within 90 days). Of the 46 patients in group 3 who did not have an EP study, however, eight died during follow-up (three during the first 90 days and none before 30 days). Furthermore, delaying EP risk stratification or ICD implantation until 3 months after surgery could, arguably, have resulted in avoidable sudden cardiac deaths.

In this study, long-term survival in patients with positive EP studies was similar to that in patients with negative EP studies. This finding may reflect the protective effect of ICD implantation in patients with positive studies, thus indicating effective risk stratification and treatment for high-risk patients. Indeed, a positive EP study was predictive of eight of nine ICD therapies delivered in group 2. However, limitations in the ability of EP studies to stratify risk in this high-risk population cannot be completely excluded.

Group 1 in this study had the worst survival, despite the presence of preoperative ICDs. The poorer survival may have been related to the greater severity of their cardiomyopathy, as manifested by larger, less contractile ventricles and the presence of a preoperative ICD (a marker for a history of or risk for life-threatening cardiac arrhythmias). Because most deaths occurred as a result of progressive myocardial failure, rather than sudden arrhythmic events, these predictors may be markers of a residual propensity to develop progressive heart failure.

The question of whether SVR increases or decreases the likelihood of ventricular arrhythmias is complex. Removal of myocardial scarring may protect from ventricular arrhythmias. However, the resultant ventriculectomy scar may be proarrhythmic. Here the rate of positive EP studies was 48 (42%) of 113, and the risk of arrhythmic events (ICD therapies plus sudden death mortality) in groups 1 and 2 was 16 (15%) of 104. Nevertheless, the overall incidence of sudden death was 1 (0.5%) of 217 by using the current strategy of early risk stratification and/or ICD implantation when feasible.

The Role of Preoperative EP Testing in Patients with LV Aneurysms Who Qualify for SVR: The Karolinska Data

In a large series by Sartipy and colleagues [44], most patients eligible for SVR underwent a preoperative EP study. In patients with spontaneous or inducible ventricular tachycardia (VT), endocardial resection and cryoablation was performed. In patients with preoperative clinical VT, an EP study before hospital discharge was performed, and in patients with inducible-only VT, they performed an EP study 3–6 months after the operation. In case of postoperative clinical or inducible VT, they recommended ICD implantation. They reported in a series of 53 consecutive patients undergoing SVR and surgical intervention for VT. The success rate in terms of VT control was 90%.

ICD firing is associated with a certain amount of discomfort for the patient. ICDs indisputably save lives, but the price can be high both in terms of money and patient well-being. Therefore, the aim must be to eliminate the need for ICD. By adding specific antiarrhythmic surgical procedures, such as endocardectomy and cryoablation, in patients undergoing SVR, there is a potentially curative treatment option. In their view, an EP study is necessary after SVR when surgical intervention for VT has been included to identify surgical failures in which ICD therapy is warranted.

In their opinion, patients scheduled for SVR should be assessed for ventricular arrhythmias, and if present, specific arrhythmia surgery should be performed concomitantly, and the postoperative result should be verified by means of EP studies. With this protocol, implantation of an ICD will not be needed in most patients after SVR including surgical intervention for VT. This is one of the large series on patients subjected to SVR which demonstrates the need for preoperative EP studies to qualify patients for adjuvant cryoablation during SVR.

Summary

The incidence of ventricular tachyarrhythmias in ischemic cardiomyopathy is linked to its pathophysiological substrate. It may originate from ventricular dilatation per se but is usually linked to the amount of scarred myocardium, usually located at the interventricular septum, forming a focus for reentry in the genesis of ventricular tachyarrhythmias. The exclusion of the septal scar with restoration of the ellipsoid ventricular geometry may be sufficient in some patients without extensive scarring where exclusion of the scar tissue is complete. However, in some patients with more extensive scarring where complete exclusion is not possible, the persistence of foci for potential reentry and ventricular tachycardia exists even after surgery. Moreover, in patients with preoperative ventricular tachycardia, the necessity for an associated cryoablation during SVR is paramount. In patients without spontaneous VT on Holter monitoring, the option of EP studies for inducibility preoperatively is entirely on the discretion of the treating physician. The postoperative patients who have undergone cryoablation require an EP study before discharge and at 6 months, and on demonstrating inducible VT, require an ICD. There are several gray zones in the management of this difficult group of patients, and management options have been individualized. This mandates clear-cut guidelines in the arrhythmia management options for this difficult subset of patients.

References

1. Cox JL. Cardiac surgery for arrhythmias. J Cardiovasc Electrophysiol. 2004;15:250–62.
2. Josephson ME. Clinical cardiac electrophysiology, techniques and Interpretations. 2nd ed. Philadelphia: Lea & Febiger; 1993. p. 436–7.
3. Bourke JP, Richards DA, Ross DL, Wallace EM, McGuire MA, Uther JB. Routine programmed electrical stimulation in survivors of acute myocardial infarction for prediction of spontaneous ventricular tachyarrhythmias during follow-up results, optimal stimulation protocol and cost-effective screening. J Am Coll Cardiol. 1991;18:780–8.
4. Wilber DJ, Olshansky B, Moran JF, Scanlon PJ. Electrophysiological testing and nonsustained ventricular tachycardia. Use and limitations in patients with coronary artery disease and impaired ventricular function. Circulation. 1990;82:350–8.
5. Babuty D, Lab MJ. Mechanoelectric contributions to sudden cardiac death. Cardiovasc Res. 2001;50:270–9.

6. St John SM, Lee D, Rouleau JL, Goldman S, Plappert T, Braunwald E, et al. Left ventricular remodeling and ventricular arrhythmias after myocardial infarction. Circulation. 2003;107(20):2577–82.
7. Foppl M, Hoffmann A, Amann FW, Roth J, Stulz P, Hasse J, et al. Sudden cardiac death after aortic valve surgery: incidence and concomitant factors. Clin Cardiol. 1989;12(4):202–7.
8. Mcgoon MD, Fuster V, Mcgoon DC, Pumphrey CW, Pluth JR, Elveback LR. Aortic and mitral valve incompetence: long-term follow-up (10 to 19 years) of patients treated with the Starr-Edwards prosthesis. J Am Coll Cardiol. 1984;3(4):930–8.
9. Michel PL, Mandagout O, Vahanian A, Cormier B, Iung B, Luxereau P, et al. Ventricular arrhythmias in aortic valve disease before and after surgery. J Heart Valve Dis. 1992;1(1):72–9.
10. Hassapoyannes CA, Stuck LM, Hornung CA, Berbin MC, Flowers NC. Effect of left ventricular aneurysm on risk of sudden and nonsudden cardiac death. Am J Cardiol. 1991;67:454–9.
11. Di Donato M, Sabatier M, Dor V, Buckberg G, and the RESTORE Group. Ventricular arrhythmias after LV remodelling: surgical ventricular restoration or ICD? Heart Fail Rev. 2004;9:299–306.
12. Marrouche NF, Verma A, Wazni O, et al. Mode of initiation and ablation of ventricular fibrillation storms in patients with ischemic cardiomyopathy. J Am Coll Cardiol. 2004;43:1715–20.
13. Bourke JP, Campbell RW, McComb JM, Furniss SS, Doig JC, Hilton CJ. Surgery for postinfarction ventricular tachycardia in the pre-implantable cardioverter defibrillator era: early and long term outcomes in 100 consecutive patients. Heart. 1999;82:156–62.
14. Stephenson LW, Hargrove 3rd WC, Ratcliffe MB, Edmunds Jr LH. Surgery for left ventricular aneurysm. Early survival with and without endocardial resection. Circulation. 1989;79(Pt 2):I108–11.
15. Kaul TK, Fields BL, Riggins LS, Wyatt DA, Jones CR. Ventricular arrhythmia following successful myocardial revascularization incidence, predictors and prevention. Eur J Cardiothorac Surg. 1998;13:629–36.
16. O'Rourke RA. Role of myocardial revascularization in sudden cardiac death. Circulation. 1992;85 Suppl 1:I112–7.
17. Dor V, Saab M, Coste P, Kornaszewska M, Montiglio F. Left ventricular aneurysm: a new surgical approach. Thorac Cardiovasc Surg. 1989;37:11–9.
18. Dor V, Sabatier M, Montiglio F, Rossi P, Toso A, Di Donato M. Results of nonguided subtotal endocardiectomy associated with left ventricular reconstruction in patients with ischemic ventricular arrhythmias. J Thorac Cardiovasc Surg. 1994;107:1301–8.
19. Rastegar H, Link MS, Foote CB, Wang PJ, Manolis AS, Estes 3rd NA. Perioperative and long-term results with mapping-guided subendocardial resection and left ventricular endoaneurysmorrhaphy. Circulation. 1996;94:1041–8.
20. Bechtel JFM, Tölg R, Graf B, Richardt G, Noetzold A, Kraatz EG, Sievers H-H, Bartels C. High incidence of sudden death late after anterior LV-aneurysm repair. Eur J Cardiothorac Surg. 2004;25:807–11.
21. Moss AJ. MADIT-II: substudies and their implications. Card Electrophysiol Rev. 2003;7(4):430–3.
22. Reynolds MR, Josephson ME. MADIT II (second Multicenter Automated Defibrillator Implantation Trial) debate: risk stratification, costs, and public policy. Circulation. 2003;108(15):1779–83.
23. Sosa E, Scanavacca M, D'avila A, Fukushima J, Jatene A. Long-term results of visually guided left ventricular reconstruction as single therapy to treat ventricular tachycardia associated with postinfarction anteroseptal aneurysm. J Cardiovasc Electrophysiol. 1998;9(11):1133–43.
24. Frapier JM, Hubaut JJ, Pasquie JL, Chaptal PA. Large encircling cryoablation without mapping for ventricular tachycardia after anterior myocardial infarction: longterm outcome. J Thorac Cardiovasc Surg. 1998;116(4):578–83.
25. Ohnishi S, Kasanuki H. Long-term outcome of pharmacological and nonpharmacological treatment for ventricular arrhythmias. J Cardiol. 2000;35 Suppl 1:75–84.
26. Athanasuleas CL, Buckberg GD, Stanley AW, Siler W, Dor V, Di Donato M, et al. Surgical ventricular restoration in the treatment of congestive heart failure due to post-infarction ventricular dilation. J Am Coll Cardiol. 2004;44(7):1439–45.
27. Di Donato M, Toso A, Dor V, et al. Surgical ventricular restoration improves mechanical intraventricular dyssynchrony in ischemic cardiomyopathy. Circulation. 2004;109:2536–43.
28. Zagrodzky JD, Ramaswamy K, Page RL, et al. Biventricular pacing decreases the inducibility of ventricular tachycardia in patients with ischemic cardiomyopathy. Am J Cardiol. 2001;87:1208–10.
29. Higgins SL, Yong P, Sheck D, et al. Biventricular pacing diminishes the need for implantable cardioverter defibrillator therapy. Ventak CHF Investigators. J Am Coll Cardiol. 2000;36:824–7.
30. Kies P, Bax JJ, Molhoek SG, et al. Effect of left ventricular remodeling after cardiac resynchronization therapy on frequency of ventricular arrhythmias. Am J Cardiol. 2004;94:130–2.
31. Breithardt OA, Stellbrink C, Herbots L, et al. Cardiac resynchronization therapy can reverse abnormal myocardial strain distribution in patients with heart failure and left bundle branch block. J Am Coll Cardiol. 2003;42:486–94.
32. Barsheshet A, Wang PJ, Moss AJ, Solomon SD, Al-Ahmad A, McNitt S, Foster E, Huang DT, Klein HU, Zareba W, Eldar M, Goldenberg I. Reverse remodeling and the risk of ventricular tachyarrhythmias in the MADIT-CRT (Multicenter Automatic Defibrillator Implantation Trial–Cardiac Resynchronization Therapy). J Am Coll Cardiol. 2011;57:2416–23.
33. Harding JD, Piacentino III V, Gaughan JP, Houser SR, Margulies KB. Electrophysiological alterations after mechanical circulatory support in patients with advanced cardiac failure. Circulation. 2001;104(11):1241–7.

34. Dor V. The treatment of refractory ischemic ventricular tachycardia by endoventricular patch plasty reconstruction of the left ventricle. Semin Thorac Cardiovasc Surg. 1997;9:146–55.
35. Ostermeyer J, Breithardt G, Borgreffe M, Godehardt E, Siepel L, Bircks W. Surgery for ventricular tachycardias: complete versus partial encircling endocardial ventriculotomy. J Thorac Cardiovasc Surg. 1984;87: 517–25.
36. Di Donato M, Toso A, Maioli M, Sabatier M, Stanley Jr AW, Dor V. Intermediate survival and predictors of death after surgical ventricular restoration. Semin Thorac Cardiovasc Surg. 2001;13:468–75.
37. Suma H, Isomura T, Horii T, Hisatomi K. Left ventriculoplasty for ischemic cardiomyopathy. Eur J Cardiothorac Surg. 2001;20:319–23.
38. Mickleborough LL. Left ventricular reconstruction for ischemic cardiomyopathy. Semin Thorac Cardiovasc Surg. 2002;14:144–9.
39. Frapier JM, Hubaut JJ, Pasquié JL, Chaptal PA. Large encircling cryoablation for ventricular tachycardia after anterior myocardial infarction: long term outcomes. J Thorac Cardiovasc Surg. 1998;116: 578–83.
40. Guiraudon GM, Thakur RK, Klein GJ, Yee R, Guiraudon CM, Sharma A. Encircling endocardial cryoablation for ventricular tachycardia after myocardial infarction: experience with 33 patients. Am Heart J. 1994;128:982–9.
41. Parachuri VR, Adhyapak SM, Kumar P, Setty S, Rathod R, Shetty DP. Ventricular restoration by linear endoventricular patchplasty and linear repair. Asian Cardiovasc Thorac Ann. 2008;16:401–6.
42. Rao Parachuri V, Adhyapak SM. Surgical cryoablation for ventricular tachycardia in patients undergoing surgical ventricular restoration: Lessons learned from radiofrequency ablation. DOI: 10.1016/j.jtcvs.2012.03.023.
43. O'Neill JO, Starling RC, Khaykin Y, McCarthy PM, Young JB, Hail M, Albert NM, Smedira N, Chung MK. Residual high incidence of ventricular arrhythmias after left ventricular reconstructive surgery. J Thorac Cardiovasc Surg. 2005;130:1250–6.
44. Sartipy U, Albåge A, Lindblom D. The Dor procedure for left ventricular reconstruction. Ten-year clinical experience. Eur J Cardiothorac Surg. 2005;27:1005–10.
45. Zipes DP, Tomaselli GF. What causes sudden death in heart failure? Circ Res. 2004;95(8):754–63.

Role of Mitral Valve Surgery in Surgical Ventricular Restoration for Left Ventricular Aneurysms

12

Introduction

In ischemic cardiomyopathy with large left ventricular aneurysms, ventricular size increases in response to the surface area of infracted scarred myocardium. This dilatation of contractile myocardium is a compensatory hemodynamic response to maintain an effective forward stroke volume and can be seen as an extension of the Frank–Starling mechanism.

The secondary changes affecting the mitral valve to cause mitral incompetence are ventricular stretch which alters leaflet coaptation, widening of the mitral annulus coinciding with a larger cardiac base, and broadening of the width between the papillary muscle bases which amplifies leaflet tethering and further limits leaflet coaptation. It has been extensively studied and proven that mitral regurgitation after a myocardial infarction significantly increases mortality. Therefore, during the planning stage of surgical ventricular restoration, interventions should be developed which will restore the altered spatial structure of ventricular size and shape with its attendant valvular perturbations back toward normal.

Definition of Ischemic Mitral Regurgitation

Chronic ischemic mitral regurgitation can be defined as mitral regurgitation occurring as a consequence of myocardial infarction or chronic myocardial ischemia in the absence of any inherent structural damage to the leaflets, chordae, or papillary muscles (PMs) [1]. According to Borger et al., it should be defined as MR occurring more than 1 week after MI, with one or more LV segmental wall motion abnormalities, significant coronary artery disease (CAD) in the territory supplying the wall motion abnormality, and structurally normal leaflets and chordae [2].

As a consequence, ventricular remodeling can lead to significant changes in the geometry of the mitral valve apparatus leading to MR. Thus, chronic ischemic mitral regurgitation is primarily caused by a disease of the LV and not by a disease of the valve itself [1, 2]. It is also often defined as functional MR or secondary MR (as opposed to structural, primary, or organic MR), which indicates that MR occurs in the absence of any inherent structural damage to the leaflets, chordae, or papillary muscles.

Prevalence of Chronic Ischemic Mitral Regurgitation

The prevalence of chronic ischemic mitral regurgitation is difficult to assess because of the heterogeneity of MR patients presented in different studies. In addition to the impact of the modality used to identify MR, discrepancies are also related to the timing of imaging [3]. Chronic ischemic mitral regurgitation occurs in approximately 20–25% of patients followed up after MI [4, 5], in 50% of patients with postinfarct congestive heart failure [5], in 11–19% of patients

V R. Parachuri, S.M. Adhyapak, *Ventricular Geometry in Post-Myocardial Infarction Aneurysms*,
DOI 10.1007/978-1-4471-2861-8_12, © Springer-Verlag London 2012

undergoing cardiac catheterization for symptomatic coronary artery disease [6], and in 28% of patients undergoing CABG [7]. Chronic ischemic mitral regurgitation is more common after inferior MI (38%) than after anterior MI (10%) at echocardiographic follow-up after 24 months [8]. Chronic ischemic mitral regurgitation may appear up to 6 weeks after MI [9]. The delay is attributed to remodeling of the LV.

The SAVE (Survival and Ventricular Enlargement) study demonstrated that mild mitral regurgitation increases the risk of cardiovascular mortality, even in patients without congestive heart failure [10]. Patients with mitral regurgitation had a higher incidence of cardiovascular mortality (29% vs 12%, $p < 0.001$) and congestive heart failure (24% vs 16%, $p < 0.001$) than patients without mitral regurgitation at a mean of 3.5 years after MI [10].

Mortality increases even when MR is mild, and there is a graded relationship between MR severity and mortality independent of LV function [11]. Grigioni et al., more recently, showed that MR is independently related to a 3.6-fold increase in the risk of congestive heart failure in patients with no or minimal symptoms [12]. These studies may differ in design, setting, and technique, but they consistently indicate that MR has an adverse prognosis with increased risk of death and congestive heart failure.

The Role of Ventricular Remodeling in Modifications of the Mitral Valve Anatomy and Mitral Regurgitation

Several anatomical substrates act in concert to produce mitral incompetence: the annulus, papillary muscles, interpapillary distance, leaflets, and chordae.

Mitral Chordae and Leaflet Tethering

Mitral valve chordae can be divided in primary and secondary chordae. Secondary chordae are the most responsible chordae for leaflet restriction in MR but are not required to prevent leaflet prolapse. Apical tenting of the mitral valve leaflets is regionally augmented in the middle portion of the anterior leaflet with basal (second-order) chordal insertion, which produces a typical anterior leaflet concavity or anterior leaflet bend (the so-called seagull sign or hockey stick configuration).

The systolic position of the leaflets is determined by two opposing forces. Transmitral pressure force (or closing force) pushes the leaflets toward the left atrium, while tethering force of the chordae pulls the leaflets toward the PMs [13, 14]. Apical displacement of the leaflets results from a greater tethering force, caused by a reduced closing force and/or an increased tethering force [13, 14]. Displacement of the PMs directly increases tethering force [13, 14]. The position of the anterior annulus is fixed at the aortic root. Therefore, the distance between the anterior annulus and the PM tips can be used as a measure of PM displacement [13]. These distances can be measured in the apical two- and four-chamber views during routine two-dimensional transthoracic echocardiography [15] (Fig. 12.7).

PM tethering is not always proportional to LV dilatation. In anteroseptal MI, there may be significant global LV remodeling without outward PM displacement and without MR [17]. In inferoposterior MI, however, there may be less global LV remodeling but more local LV remodeling with significant PM displacement and significant MR [8, 17]. Thus, MR is proportional to the outward displacement of the PMs rather than to global LV dilatation [13]. Consequently, two types of leaflet tethering occur in MR. Symmetric tethering results from global LV remodeling with apical displacement of both PMs [18]. This generally produces a central MR jet. Asymmetric tethering results from regional LV remodeling with displacement of the posteromedial PM and systolic posterior leaflet restriction [18]. This generally produces an eccentric MR jet directed toward the posterior left atrial wall. However, it is controversial whether asymmetric PM displacement leads to asymmetric tethering. Approximately, symmetric leaflet tethering can occur in inferior MI with potential asymmetric PM displacement [19].

Influence of LV Force of Contraction

Reduced closing force due to LV dysfunction can increase MR in the presence of increased tethering force due to PM displacement [20]. LV dysfunction without LV dilatation and mitral valve tethering fails to produce significant MR [21]. Interestingly, Schwammenthal et al. showed that the severity of MR dynamically changes within a cardiac cycle, with the severity maximal in early and late systole and minimal in midsystole with maximal LV pressure (also known as the "loitering pattern") [22].

Papillary Muscle Dysfunction

PM dysfunction (syndrome) was first described as the main cause of MR [22, 23]; however, this could not be confirmed. In the leaflet tethering theory, the effect of PM dysfunction can be twofold. LV remodeling in the wall close to the PM may result in increased tethering [24]. In this case, PM dysfunction increases tethering [24]. On the other hand, when LV remodeling occurs in the wall close to the PM and extends to include the PM, PM dysfunction may decrease longitudinal PM shortening and tethering [24, 25]. This may even cause leaflet prolapse [26]. In addition, PM dyssynchrony can potentially worsen MR [27, 28].

Annular Dilatation

Although annular dilatation is often associated with LV dilatation in MR, it is at this point unclear whether annular dilatation is a major determinant of MR in the absence of leaflet tethering due to LV dilatation. Annular dilatation as an isolated lesion is suggested to be insufficient to cause significant MR [29]. Annular dilatation may, however, as a modulating factor, influence MR in the presence of leaflet tethering.

In addition, flattening of the physiological annular saddle shape in dilated ventricles can lead to increased tethering and development of MR [28, 29]. A reduced systolic contraction of the annulus can also contribute to the development of MR.

The analysis of the mitral annulus dimensions in ischemic dilated cardiomyopathy is of paramount importance in understanding the genesis of valvular dysfunction. It is assumed that the valvular dysfunction observed in these patients is related to dilation of the left ventricle (LV) and left atrium, mitral annular dilation, tearing of the chordae tendineae, and abnormal papillary muscle and LV wall contraction [30].

Valvular regurgitation in patients with ischemic or idiopathic dilated cardiomyopathy is a predictive factor of poor prognosis [31] and a frequent complication at the final stage of cardiomyopathy, contributing to aggravation of heart failure and leading to unfavorable progression [32].

Echocardiographic analysis in patients with dilated cardiomyopathy with and without mitral regurgitation has demonstrated that dilation of the mitral annulus occurs only in some patients and is not proportional to the degree of LV dilation. Thus, valvular regurgitation associated with LV dilation has a mechanism of dilation independent of that of the mitral annulus, such as loss of sphincter action of the annulus or poor alignment of the papillary muscles [33]. Anatomic studies of the mitral annulus in hearts from patients with dilated cardiomyopathy and in normal hearts have demonstrated that mitral dilation alone is usually not responsible for valvular regurgitation. There must be also a deformation in the fibrous skeleton to dilate the annulus and cause valvular regurgitation [34]. Observations in LV experimental models have shown that mitral regurgitation occurs only when the annulus is more than 1.75-fold more dilated or 1.50-fold dilated with an apical displacement of the posterolateral papillary muscle, indicating that the mitral valve compensates for annular dilation because of the wide surface of its leaflets [35]. Knowledge of mitral valvular apparatus alterations can be applied to improve several surgical repair techniques involving the annulus, leaflets, chordae tendineae, and papillary muscles, together or separately, thus justifying its anatomic study in ischemic dilated cardiomyopathy [27, 36].

Alexandre Ciappina Hueb and coworkers studied the mitral valve apparatus in patients with idiopathic dilated cardiomyopathy and ischemic cardiomyopathy by echocardiography and postmortem pathological studies [37]. Mitral insufficiency is common in patients with ischemic and idiopathic dilated cardiomyopathy. Although the real mechanism of functional insufficiency has not been completely understood, one could suppose that some concurrent factors, such as displacement of the papillary muscles, valvular insertion traction in the fibrous annulus, and decreased contractile force in the LV leading to decreased transvalvular pressure, are among the probable etiologic factors [13].

Anatomic studies have demonstrated that mitral annular dilation rarely causes regurgitation [66]. Therefore, there must be some abnormality in the fibrous skeleton of the heart to make the annulus dilate and cause mitral regurgitation. The mitral annulus comprises two fibrous structures—the right and left fibrous trigones—that are in an anterior position. However, its posterior segment has no fibrous structures that could theoretically be dilated.

The mitral annulus is a dynamic structure that undergoes changes in shape and size of all its segments, both in the posterior and anterior portions during the various phases of the cardiac cycle. The dynamics of the anterior leaflet thus could be a much more active component in the mitral valve apparatus.

Kunzelman and colleagues [38] compared the mitral valve perimeter and the extension of the insertion of each leaflet in situ and after excision of the valve and observed increases by 31% in posterior leaflet insertion and by 3.3% in the anterior leaflet insertion when leaflets were excised.

Hueb et al. analyzed seven mitral annular variables to check the behavior of the annulus in ischemic and idiopathic dilated cardiomyopathy: perimeter, area, leaflet area, fibrous and muscular portions of the annulus, and insertion perimeters of the anterior and posterior leaflets.

The increases of mitral valve area and leaflet area that were observed in ischemic and idiopathic dilated cardiomyopathy occurred in a linear pattern (Fig. 12.1). Therefore, they concluded that a compensatory mechanism of the leaflets exists related to their own condition of natural redundancy. This mechanism compensates for mitral regurgitation when the dilation of the ring occurs. According to many authors [39, 40], the short perimeter distance between fibrous trigones is an area that could not be distended, because it is part of the fibrous heart skeleton. This study compared normal hearts with hearts with dilated cardiomyopathy and demonstrated a proportional increase in the fibrous and muscular portions of the annulus relative to the degree of dilation of the mitral annulus. Because the fibrous portion involved only 21.5% of the mitral circumference, they also measured the insertion perimeter of the anterior leaflet, which involved 43% of the circumference. Both measures, the shorter perimeter distance between fibrous trigones representing the fibrous portion of the annulus and the insertion perimeter of the anterior leaflet, showed an increase proportional to that observed in the valvular annulus. These data are in disagreement with the literature, in which most reports do not consider the fibrous portion of the annulus to be increased [41], and with data from the authors previously cited [42, 43], who accept a minimal increase.

They recommended that as the dilation also occurs in the anterior portion of the ring in hearts with ischemic or idiopathic dilated cardiomyopathy, the use of complete mitral annuloplasty techniques over partial annuloplasty aligned to the posterior annulus.

Kono et al. [44] studied the effects of ventricular geometry, mitral annular geometry, and underlying wall motion abnormalities in the development of functional mitral regurgitation in ischemic cardiomyopathy.

The onset of functional mitral regurgitation during the course of evolving heart failure is associated with changes in left ventricular shape manifested by increased chamber sphericity. Neither mitral annulus dilatation, left ventricular chamber enlargement, nor abnormalities in ventricular wall motion were present when mitral regurgitation first manifested. Therefore, they concluded that these anatomical changes were not integral in the development of functional mitral regurgitation. The transformation of left ventricular shape was the primary determinant of functional mitral regurgitation.

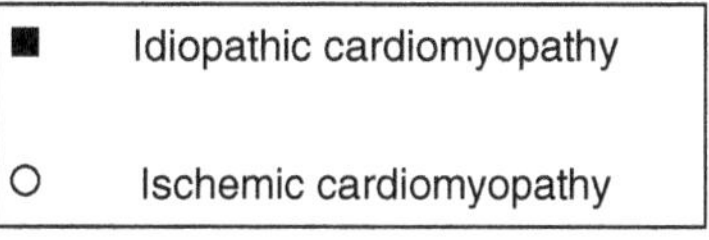

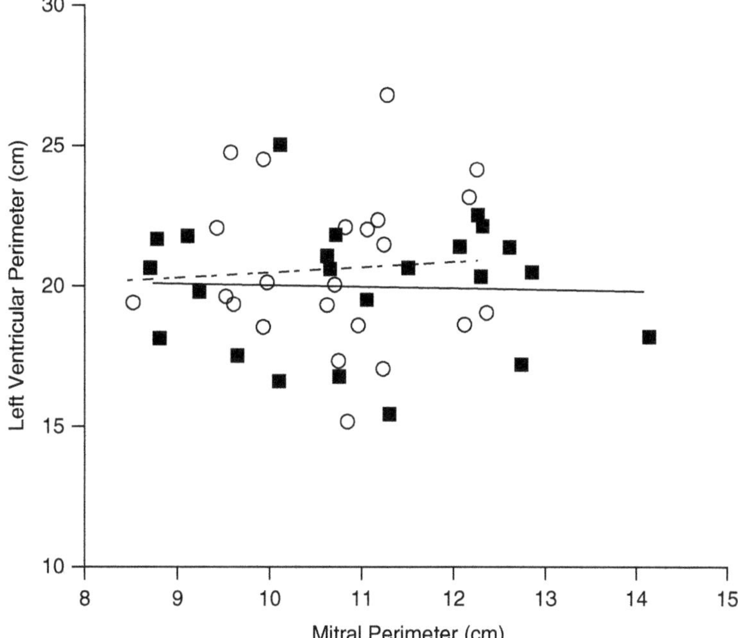

Fig. 12.1 Progressive increases in LV perimeter and mitral valve perimeter were observed when normal hearts and hearts with ischemic or idiopathic DCM were compared. In linear regression, it was observed in hearts with both ischemic and idiopathic DCM that LV perimeter was not linearly proportional with mitral valve perimeter. That is, the degree of LV dilation was not related to that of mitral annular dilation. LV and mitral annular perimeters in ischemic and idiopathic DCM (With permission from Hueb et al. [37]. Copyright Elsevier)

Here the onset of mitral regurgitation was associated with an increase in the perpendicular distance between the mitral annulus plane and the coaptation point of the mitral valve leaflets. An increase in this distance indicates retraction of the mitral valve leaflets toward the ventricular apex leading to incomplete mitral valve closure during systole.

In the normally ellipsoid left ventricle, the position of the papillary muscles permits their contraction to exert a vertical force on the chordae tendineae. Application of this force moves the mitral valve leaflets together during isovolumetric contraction and restrains their motion during ventricular ejection.

In a more spherical ventricle, the papillary muscles may undergo lateral migration and therefore may not be vertically aligned with the mitral annulus. In this situation, the forces exerted on the leaflets through the chordae tendineae become more lateral than vertical. This lateral tension prevents apposition of the leaflets and renders the valve incompetent Fig. 12.2.

The progression of mitral regurgitation with heart failure was studied in the canine model, and the development of profound ventricular dysfunction at 3 months was associated with worsening of mitral regurgitation. Here there was progressive increase in left ventricular sphericity, increase in mitral annular dimensions, increase in left ventricular chamber dimensions, and increase in wall motion abnormalities overlying the papillary muscles. For progression of mitral regurgitation, all these factors may act in concert to worsen the existing mitral regurgitation. However, the development of functional mitral regurgitation requires increase in left ventricular sphericity as the substrate.

A finite element model study of ischemic MR in sheep has thrown light on the mechanisms involved in generation of ischemic MR [45]. The increased infarct stiffness had a beneficial effect

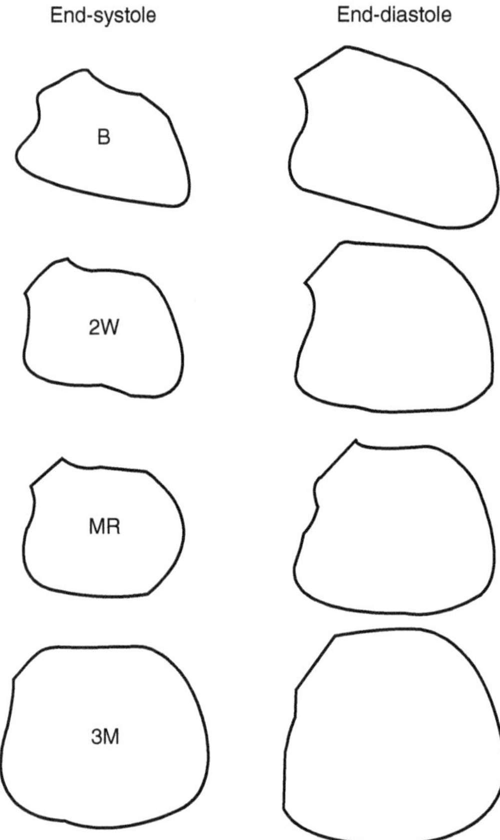

Fig. 12.2 End systolic (*left*) and end diastolic (*right*) left ventricular silhouettes from a study dog. The silhouettes depict the changes in LV shape at baseline (*B*), at 2 weeks before (*2W*), at the time of onset of mitral regurgitation (*MR*) and at 3 months (*3M*) after the onset of functional mitral regurgitation (With permission from Kono et al. [44])

on papillary muscle tethering and MR. Similar to clinical studies, it was found that the severity of MR correlated positively with the gap between the anterior and posterior mitral leaflets which occurred due to leaflet tethering.

Hemodynamic Consequences of Ischemic Mitral Regurgitation

The increase in preload caused by MR after MI is not accompanied by a parallel increase in contractility [46]. The chronic volume overload in a ventricle that has decreased compliance causes an increase in wall stress and left atrial (LA), ventricular end-diastolic, and wedge pressures. The left atrium (LA) and ventricle enlarge, resulting in pulmonary hypertension and congestion, leading ultimately to heart failure and death [47, 48]. Ventricular dilatation increases tethering, which worsens MR severity, creating a cycle whereby MR begets MR in a self-perpetuating manner [49].

Evaluation of Ischemic Mitral Regurgitation by 2-D Echocardiography

Several parameters can be measured to evaluate the severity and pattern of mitral valve tethering. Tenting area (TA) (the area between the tented leaflets and the annular plane in systole) and tenting height (TH) (distance between the point of leaflet coaptation and the mitral annular plane in systole) show a strong and positive correlation with the effective regurgitant orifice.

Apart from providing additional information on tethering severity and pattern, measurement of parameters such as TA, TH, posterior and anterior leaflet tethering angles (PTA and ATA), and interpapillary muscle distance (IPMD) has been shown to provide prognostic information about the surgical treatment results of MR.

Surgical Ventricular Restoration with Concomitant Mitral Regurgitation

To determine the effect of SVR on mitral regurgitation, Prucz et al. [50] studied two cohorts of patients with MR who underwent CABG and SVR.

Revascularization with concomitant SVR and mitral valve repair has been shown to improve left ventricular and mitral valve function [51–53]. However, the question of the effect of SVR on mitral valve regurgitation independent of mitral valve procedures was undertaken.

Any comparison between SVR+CABG and CABG groups can be difficult. Previous studies have achieved such comparisons by classifying CABG patients with an increased left ventricular internal diastolic dimension (6.0 cm) as SVR candidates [54]. However, not all bypass patients with a dilated heart due to ischemic cardiomyopathy are eligible for the SVR procedure. There was no significant difference in preoperative MR grade between the two groups. However, postoperatively, patients undergoing SVR with CABG were more likely to have an improvement in MR grade with a significant number of patients improving to 0 to 1+ MR.

Menicanti and colleagues [51] showed that in patients with a preoperative MR grade of 2.9 ± 1.2 who underwent SVR + CABG with mitral repair, MR improved to 1.5 ± 1.2 late after surgery. These patients also had significant improvement in EF (0.30–0.34) and NYHA functional class. Additionally, this group showed that 87% of patients with 3+ to 4+ MR preoperatively who underwent only SVR + CABG had 1+ to 2+ MR postoperatively. Based on their studies, the group concluded that 2+ MR was detrimental and recommended that even mild MR be corrected. In this study, in the SVR + CABG cohort, the average MR grade improved from 2.24 ± 0.5 to 1.24 ± 0.9, with 60% of patients improving to 0 to 1+ MR. At follow-up, left ventricular function, NYHA functional class, and incidence for rehospitalization for congestive heart failure were all significantly improved in the SVR + CABG group. It therefore appears that in some patients with 2+ to 3+ MR, SVR + CABG without mitral valve repair may have results comparable with SVR + CABG with mitral valve repair.

The SVR procedure most likely improves MR by reducing chordal tethering and improving left ventricular geometry. Yu and colleagues [55] showed that an increase in left ventricular end-systolic volume is associated with an increase in the interpapillary distance and distance from the anterior mitral annulus to the medial papillary muscle root. During the SVR procedure, the longitudinal axis is shortened by bringing the stretched papillary muscles toward the annulus to reduce the sphericity of the left ventricle thereby reducing ventricular volumes. In the series by Menicanti and colleagues, ventricular size and shape improved in patients undergoing SVR, along with reductions in chordal tethering and interpapillary muscle distance. Other studies documenting improved MR after SVR have proposed similar theories [56]. One must be careful to remember that improper placement of the purse-string or "Fontan" stitch too close to the papillary muscles can have detrimental effects and increase tethering of the subvalvular apparatus. Maintaining recognition of this issue in placing the purse string, the use of sizing devices, and the use of patches to reconstruct the ventricle can all reduce the incidence of this problem. Additionally, it is important to note that the SVR procedure does not address the annular dilation component of MR; therefore, for these patients, annular reduction may be needed.

Factors Influencing Mitral Regurgitation After Endoventricular Circular Patch Plasty

The geometric correlates of late mitral regurgitation following EVCPP and the effect of regional left ventricular deformation contributing to late mitral regurgitation in these patients was studied by Barletta et al. [57]. This was undertaken as many patients undergoing EVCPP without preoperative MR developed MR 1 year after SVR.

Wall motion was analyzed in terms of centerline fractional shortening, and LV volumes calculated according to Chapman, as previously described [58]. The shortening fraction of 90 chords, from the aortic corner (chord 1) to the mitral plane (chord 90), was obtained by dividing the systolic shortening of each chord by the end-diastolic LV perimeter to compensate for differences in size [59] and graphically reported in terms of Z value, that is, the standard deviations of mean normal shortening fraction. Akinesia was identified by Z value of fractional shortening of two or more consecutive chords of −2 or less.

Global LV shape was evaluated by calculating the eccentricity index [60] and the circular shape index [61] of end-diastolic and end-systolic LV

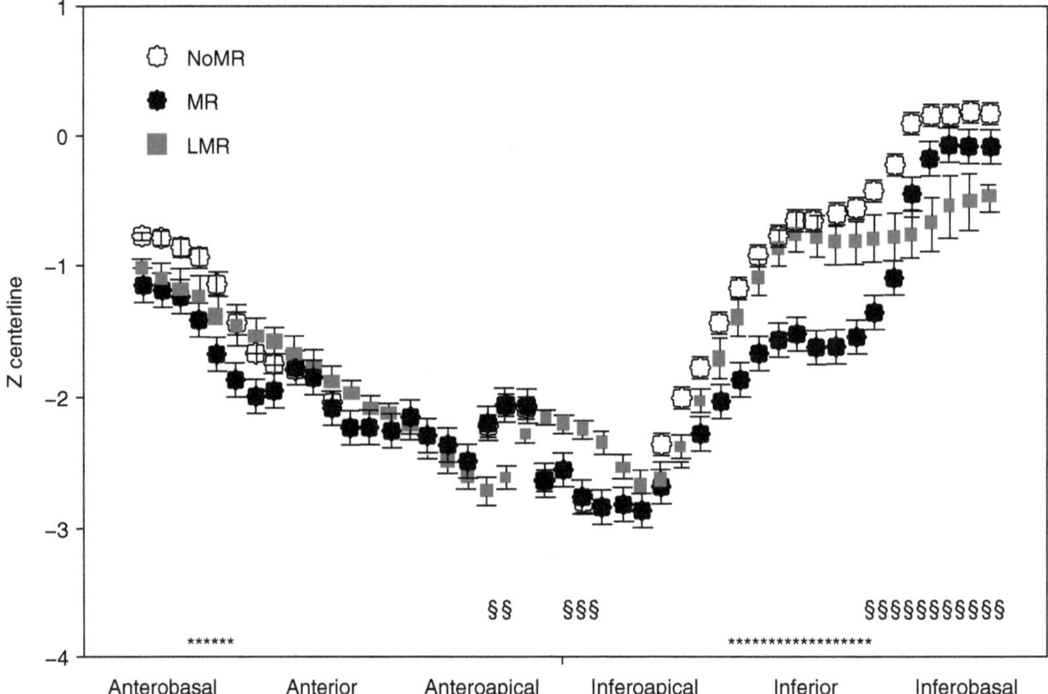

Fig. 12.3 Preoperative wall motion analysis (centerline method). The plot shows the *Z* values (mean ± SE) of fractional shortening along the left ventricular (LV) perimeter, from the aortic corner to the mitral plane. The symbol * marks the LV zones of statistical differences in wall motion between mitral regurgitation (*MR*) patients (*solid circles*) and no MR (*No MR*) patients (*open circles*). The symbol marks the LV zones of statistical differences in wall motion between late MR (*LMR*) patients (*squares*) and No MR patients (With permission from Barletta et al. [57]. Copyright Elsevier)

contours in the RAO projection. The eccentricity index, according to an ellipsoidal model, takes into account the major and the minor axes of the left ventricle and ranges between 1 (ellipse) and 0 (circle), while the circular index represents the ratio of the original shape to that of a circle, ranging between 1 (circle) and 0 (straight line).

Regional LV shape was quantitatively evaluated by measuring the regional curvature (namely, the reciprocal of the radius of the circle that best fits a segment of the arc centered at any point) that was calculated by means of a windowed Fourier series approximation of contours, in which the number of harmonics and the filter window are chosen locally to minimize the reconstruction errors and maximize the smoothness of the curve [62].

The variables that would differentiate among patients without preoperative MR those who will and those who will not have late MR were analysed. Two key factors had statistical significance: asynergy and deformation of the inferobasal region of the left ventricle (Figs. 12.3, 12.4, 12.5, 12.6, and 12.7), and high values of capillary wedge pressure. The myocardial band theory may help explain the functional importance of preoperative shape and asynergy of the inferobasal region in the development of MR after ventricular restoration surgery. The LV inferolateral region belongs to the basal circumferential loop of the myocardial band; however, it should be the site where the basal loop continues into the descending loop. Such a continuity may explain the functional and morphologic impairment of a region remote from the ischemic damage. The link between asynergy and deformation of the inferobasal region and late MR can be identified in the interference between the circumferentially arranged myocardial fibers of ventricular origin that insert into the posterior

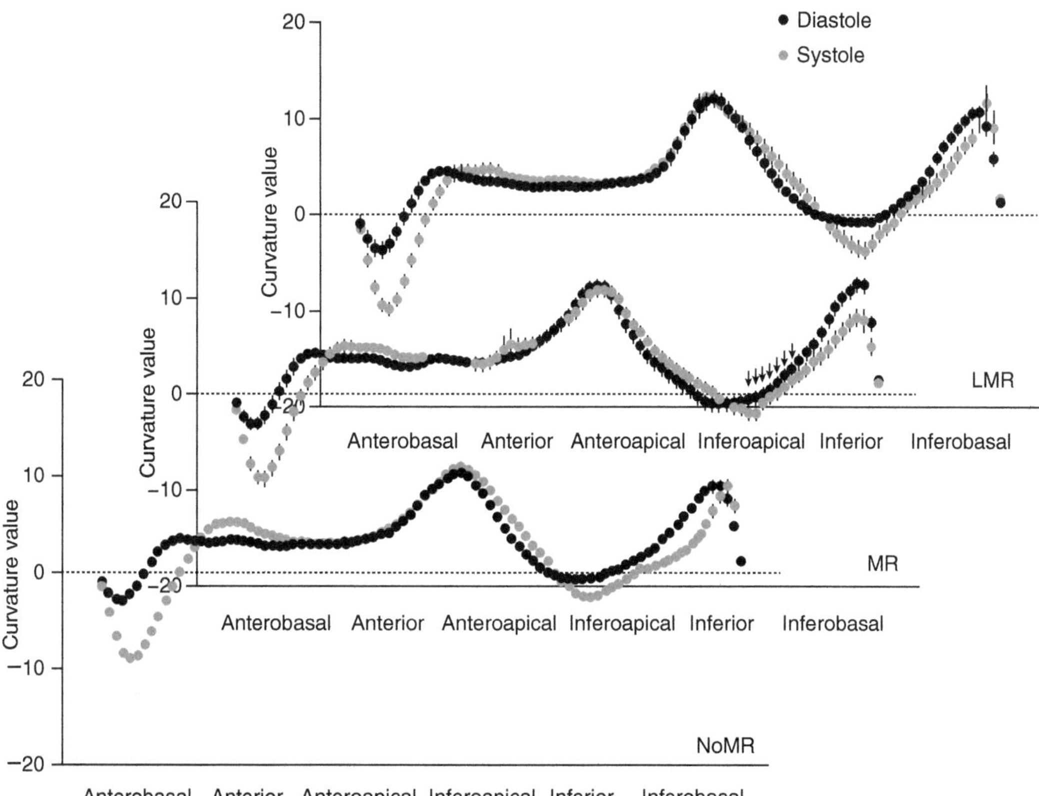

Fig. 12.4 Regional curvature analysis. Graphs are reported on three parallel planes: on each plane, systolic (*gray circles*) and diastolic (*black circles*) curvature values (mean ± SE) are plotted along the left ventricular (*LV*) perimeter, from the aortic corner to the mitral plane, for no mitral regurgitation (*NoMR*) patients in the front plane, for MR patients in the intermediate plane, and for late MR (*LMR*) patients in the back plane. *Arrows* indicate the area where systolic shape changes are different in NoMR patients in comparison with *MR* patients (two-way analysis of variance for repeated measures). The negative curvature of the inferior wall of NoMR patients significantly increased, whereas it was unchanged in MR patients (With permission from Barletta et al. [57]. Copyright Elsevier)

muscular component of the mitral annulus and the systolic contraction of the annulus itself.

The complexity of the interplay is even bigger because impaired annulus contraction not only is dependent on but also causes abnormal function of the basal LV regions. In this scenario, preexisting high capillary wedge pressure may contribute to MR development by hampering the closure kinetics of the mitral leaflets owing to a reduced driving pressure (where driving pressure equals LV systolic pressure minus left atrial systolic pressure) [13]; thus, it also may interfere with left atrium function and consequently with the presystolic annulus shrinkage [63]. Far from being just speculations, the preoperative identification of key elements able to trigger the possible development of functional MR in patients scheduled for surgical ventricular reconstruction could guide both the surgical and postoperative therapeutic strategy.

Fallacies of LV Restoration Techniques Responsible for Late MR

The technique of left ventricular restoration has a definite impact on the occurrence of MR postoperatively. It has already been discussed as to how the technique of EVCPP leads to late MR in a few patients. The use of Fontan suture and subsequent

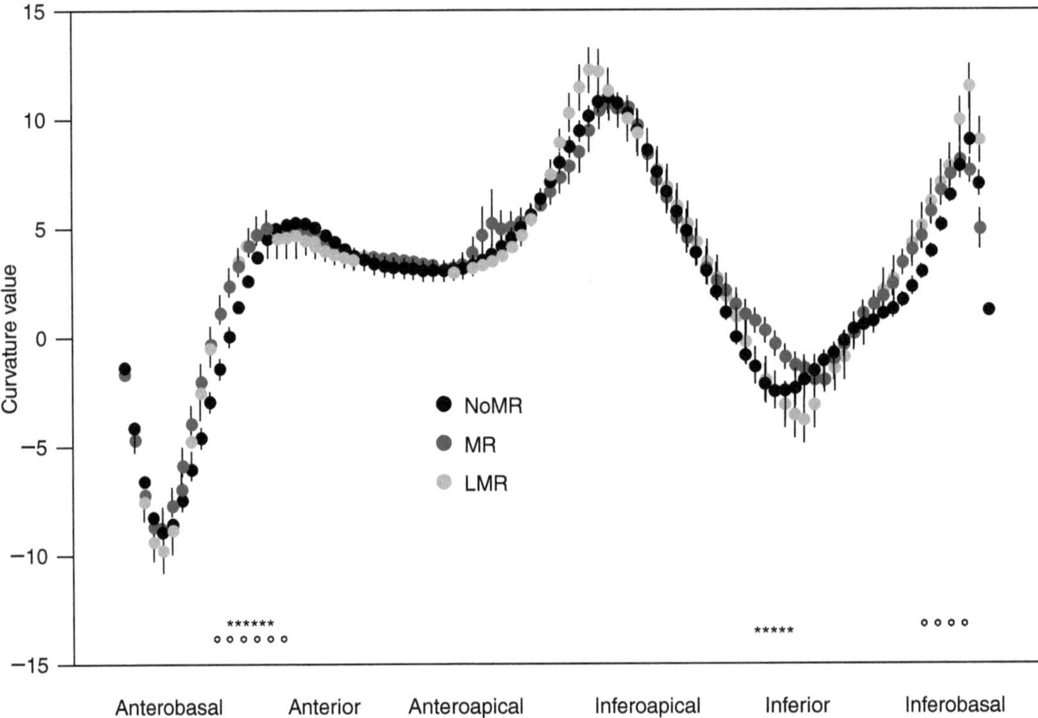

Fig. 12.5 Systolic curvature values (mean ± SE) of no mitral regurgitation (*NoMR*) patients (*black circles*), *MR* patients (*dark gray circles*), and late MR (*LMR*) patients (*light gray circles*), graphically reported along the left ventricular (*LV*) perimeter from the aortic corner to the mitral plane. The symbols * and o indicate the zones with statistically different curvature values, with respect to *NoMR* patients, of MR and LMR patients, respectively (With permission from Barletta et al. [57]. Copyright Elsevier)

plication to create a neck around the excluded infarct can lead to apical displacement of the leaflet coaptation causing late mitral regurgitation. Besides, the Fontan suture leads to persistence of LV sphericity, although the LV chamber volume is decreased which again leads to worsening MR at long term with associated re-remodeling. To overcome these complications of late occurrence of mitral regurgitation, Menicanti and colleagues [64] employed the technique of papillary muscle repositioning which involves placement of the Fontan suture in an orthogonal orientation to the mitral plane. On snaring the suture, it imbricated the bases of the papillary muscles and thereby reduced the distance between them, and decreased the left ventricular volume. There was reduction in the grade of mitral regurgitation in all but four patients. This complex surgical technique has been added as an adjunct to address the mitral regurgitation which was not addressed in totality by the EVCPP technique of SVR.

Our Data of Mitral Regurgitation in Patients Undergoing Surgical Ventricular Restoration by the EVLPP Technique

In our patients, we have used rigid restrictive Carpentier–Edwards mitral annuloplasty ring for patients with preoperative MR of 2+. The MR has decreased postoperatively to 1+ to 0 [65]. In patients with significant preoperative MR, the magnitude of LV dilatation as quantified by the EDVI was significantly greater than those without significant preoperative MR. These patients had more significant adverse ventricular remodeling warranting concomitant mitral valve annuloplasty.

None of our patients with no preoperative MR has developed MR postoperatively. We do not advocate plication of the LV by any means for reasons cited above. Therefore, we have

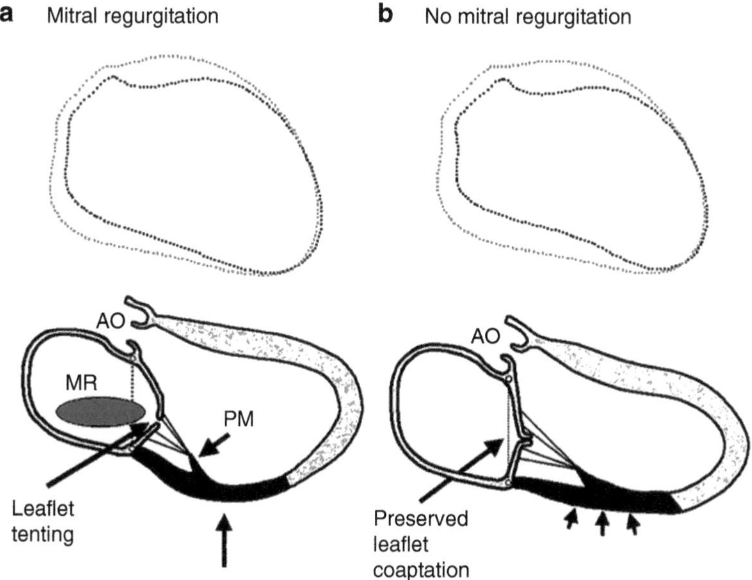

Fig. 12.6 Mechanism of negative systolic curvature. On the *top row*: mean diastolic (*gray dots*) and systolic (*black dots*) ventricular contours of mitral regurgitation (*MR*) patients (**a**) and no MR patients (**b**) were reconstructed by Fourier shape analysis (24 harmonics) by using the average spectrum of each group in comparison. The shape difference between the two groups is well apparent. On the *bottom row*: a scheme illustrating how the presence of a negative systolic curvature of the inferior wall (**b**—*short arrows*) preserves mitral leaflet coaptation, while its absence (i.e., positive curvature; **a**—*upward vertical arrow*) tethers the papillary muscle (*PM*) and tents mitral leaflets promoting MR (*AO* aorta) (With permission from Barletta et al. [57]. Copyright Elsevier)

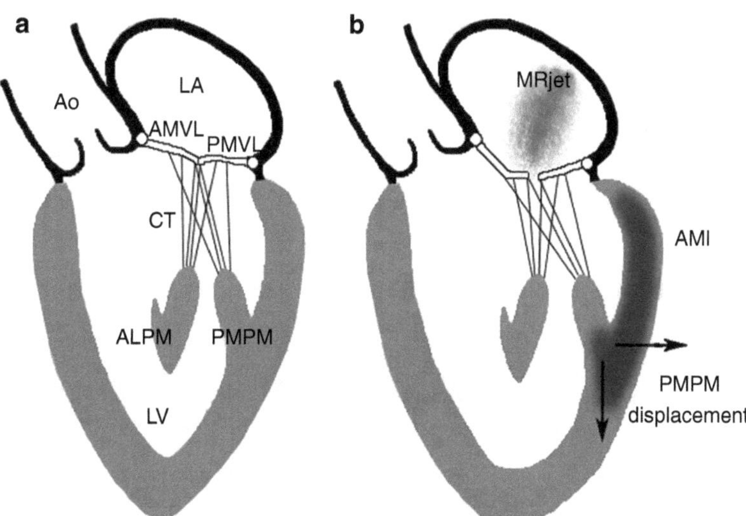

Fig. 12.7 Mechanisms of chronic ischemic mitral regurgitation (CIMR). (**a**) Normal mitral valve: the leaflets coapt at the level of or just below the mitral valve annular plane. (**b**) Mitral valve tethering: myocardial infarction leads to left ventricular remodeling, which causes apical and lateral displacement of the papillary muscles and tethering of the leaflets. Restricted systolic leaflet motion displaces the point of coaptation apically relative to the annulus which results in mitral valve tenting. Note the regionally augmented tenting in the middle portion of the anterior leaflet with basal (second-order) chordal insertion, which produces a typical anterior leaflet bend (the so-called seagull sign or hockey stick configuration). *ALPM* anterolateral papillary muscle, *AMI* area of myocardial infarction, *AMVL* anterior mitral valve leaflet, *Ao* aorta, *CT* chordae tendinae, *LA* left atrium, *LV* left ventricle, *MRjet* mitral regurgitant jet, *PMPM* posteromedian papillary muscle and *PMVL* posterior mitral valve leaflet (With permission from Bouma et al. [16]. Copyright Elsevier)

abandoned the Fontan suture. Our LV restoration by the EVLPP has shown significant beneficial LV remodeling which continued at long term. The LV when restored by use of a linear rectangular endoventricular patch ensures near-total infarct exclusion and realignment of the anterior, anterolateral, and inferior walls to a more ellipsoid geometry. The realignment of the uninfarcted portions of the anterior, anterolateral, and inferior left ventricular walls decreases the interpapillary muscle distance and realigns them, thereby inhibiting leaflet tethering and mitral regurgitation. This prevented the occurrence of late MR in those patients with no preoperative MR. The technique of EVLPP resulted in a more ellipsoid LV, obviating the need for papillary muscle imbrications. In more dilated ventricles, there was requirement for a restrictive Carpentier–Edwards mitral annuloplasty ring which decreased postoperative mitral regurgitation by effective reduction of the mitral annulus and restoration of the ellipsoid left ventricular geometry by the linear endoventricular patch plasty. There was further continued long-term reverse ventricular remodeling in all our patients which decreased the degree of mitral regurgitation from that at baseline.

References

1. Gorman RC, Gorman 3rd JH, Edmunds Jr LH. Ischemic mitral regurgitation. In: Cohn LH, Edmunds Jr LH, editors. Cardiac surgery in the adult. New York: McGraw-Hill; 2003. p. 751–69.
2. Borger MA, Alam A, Murphy PM, Doenst T, David TE. Chronic ischemic mitral regurgitation: repair, replace or rethink? Ann Thorac Surg. 2006;81:1153–61.
3. Magne J, Sénéchal M, Dumesnil JG, Pibarot P. Ischemic mitral regurgitation: a complex multifaceted disease. Cardiology. 2008;112:244–59.
4. Birnbaum Y, Chamoun AJ, Conti VR, Uretsky BF. Mitral regurgitation following acute myocardial infarction. Coron Artery Dis. 2002;13:337–44.
5. Trichon BH, Felker GM, Shaw LK, Cabell CH, O'Conner CM. Relation of frequency and severity of mitral regurgitation to survival among patients with left ventricular systolic dysfunction and heart failure. Am J Cardiol. 2003;91:538–43.
6. Hickey MS, Smith LR, Muhlbaier LH, Harrell Jr FE, Reves JG, Hinohara T, Califf RM, Pryor DB, Rankin JS. Current prognosis of ischemic mitral regurgitation: implications for future management. Circulation. 1988;78:I51–9.
7. Wierup P, Nielsen SL, Egeblad H, Scherstén H, Kimblad PO, Bech-Hansen O, Roijer A, Nilsson F, Nielsen PH, Poulsen SH, Mølgaard H. The prevalence of moderate mitral regurgitation in patients undergoing CABG. Scand Cardiovasc J. 2009;43:46–9.
8. Kumanohoso T, Otsuji Y, Yoshifuku S, Matsukida K, Koriyama C, Kisanuki A, Minagoe S, Levine RA, Tei C. Mechanism of higher incidence of ischemic mitral regurgitation in patients with inferior myocardial infarction: quantitative analysis of left ventricular and mitral valve geometry in 103 patients with prior myocardial infarction. J Thorac Cardiovasc Surg. 2003;125:135–43.
9. Filsoufi F, Salzberg SP, Adams DH. Current management of ischemic mitral regurgitation. Mt Sinai J Med. 2005;72:105–15.
10. Lamas GA, Mitchell GF, Flaker GC, Smith Jr SC, Gersh BJ, Basta L, Moyé L, Braunwald E, Pfeffer MA. Clinical significance of mitral regurgitation after acute myocardial infarction. Survival and ventricular enlargement investigators. Circulation. 1997;96:827–33.
11. Grigioni F, Enriquez-Sarano M, Zehr KJ, Bailey KR, Tajik AJ. Ischemic mitral regurgitation: long-term outcome and prognostic implications with quantitative Doppler assessment. Circulation. 2001;103:1759–64.
12. Grigioni F, Detaint D, Avierinos JF, Scott C, Tajik J, Enriquez-Sarano M. Contribution of ischemic mitral regurgitation to congestive heart failure after myocardial infarction. J Am Coll Cardiol. 2005;45:260–7.
13. He S, Fontaine AA, Schwammenthal E, Yoganathan AP, Levine RA. Integrated mechanism for functional mitral regurgitation: leaflet restriction versus coapting force: in vitro studies. Circulation. 1997;96:1826–34.
14. Otsuji Y, Levine RA, Takeuchi M, Sakata R, Tei C. Mechanism of ischemic mitral regurgitation. J Cardiol. 2008;51:145–56.
15. Yiu SF, Enriquez-Sarano M, Tribouilloy C, Seward JB, Tajik AJ. Determinants of the degree of functional mitral regurgitation in patients with systolic left ventricular dysfunction: a quantitative clinical study. Circulation. 2000;102:1400–6.
16. Bouma W, van der Horst IC, Wijdh-den Hamer IJ, Erasmus ME, Zijlstra F, Mariani MA, Ebels T. Chronic ischaemic mitral regurgitation. Current treatment results and new mechanism-based surgical approaches. Eur J Cardiothorac Surg. 2010;37:170–85.
17. Gorman 3rd JH, Gorman RC, Plappert T, Jackson BM, Hiramatsu Y, St John-Sutton MG, Edmunds Jr LH. Infarct size and location determine development of mitral regurgitation in the sheep model. J Thorac Cardiovasc Surg. 1998;115:615–22.
18. Agricola E, Oppizzi M, Maisano F, De Bonis M, Schinkel AF, Torracca L, Margonato A, Melisurgo G, Alfieri O. Echocardiographic classification of chronic ischemic mitral regurgitation caused by restricted motion according to tethering pattern. Eur J Echocardiogr. 2004;5:326–34.
19. Watanabe N, Ogasawara Y, Yamaura Y, Yamamoto K, Wada N, Kawamoto T, Toyota E, Akasaka T, Yoshida K. Geometric differences of the mitral valve tenting

between anterior and inferior myocardial infarction with significant ischemic mitral regurgitation: quantitation by novel software system with transthoracic real-time three-dimensional echocardiography. J Am Soc Echocardiogr. 2006;19:71–5.
20. Kaul S, Spotnitz WD, Glasheen WP, Touchstone DA. Mechanism of ischemic mitral regurgitation: an experimental evaluation. Circulation. 1991;84:2167–80.
21. Otsuji Y, Handschumacher MD, Liel-Cohen N, Tanabe H, Jiang L, Schwammenthal E, Guerrero JL, Nicholls LA, Vlahakes GJ, Levine RA. Mechanism of ischemic mitral regurgitation with segmental left ventricular dysfunction: three-dimensional echocardiographic studies in models of acute and chronic progressive regurgitation. J Am Coll Cardiol. 2001;37:641–8.
22. Burch GE, De Pasquale NP, Philips JH. Clinical manifestations of papillary muscle dysfunction. Arch Intern Med. 1963;112:112–7.
23. Burch GE, De Pasquale NP, Philips JH. The syndrome of papillary muscle dysfunction. Am Heart J. 1968;75:399–415.
24. Messas E, Guerrero JL, Handschumacher MD, Chow CM, Sullivan S, Schwammenthal E, Levine RA. Paradoxic decrease in ischemic mitralregurgitation with papillary muscle dysfunction: insights from three-dimensional and contrast echocardiography with strain rate measurement. Circulation. 2001;104:1952–7.
25. Uemura T, Otsuji Y, Nakashiki K, Yoshifuku S, Maki Y, Yu B, Mizukami N, Kuwahara E, Hamasaki S, Biro S, Kisanuki A, Minagoe S, Levine RA, Tei C. Papillary muscle dysfunction attenuates ischemic mitral regurgitation in patients with localized basal inferior left ventricular remodeling: insights from tissue Doppler strain imaging. J Am Coll Cardiol. 2005;46:113–9.
26. Jouan J, Tapia M, Cook RC, Lansac E, Acar C. Ischemic mitral valve prolapse: mechanisms and implications for valve repair. Eur J Cardiothorac Surg. 2004;26:1112–7.
27. Kanzaki H, Bazaz R, Schwartzman D, Dohi K, Sade LE, Gorcsan 3rd J. A mechanism for immediate reduction in mitral regurgitation after cardiac resynchronization therapy: insights from mechanical activation strain mapping. J Am Coll Cardiol. 2004;44:1619–25.
28. Ypenburg C, Lancellotti P, Tops LF, Bleeker GB, Holman ER, Piérard LA, Schalij MJ, Bax JJ. Acute effects of initiation and withdrawal of cardiac resynchronization therapy on papillary muscle dyssynchrony and mitral regurgitation. J Am Coll Cardiol. 2007;50:2071–7.
29. Otsuji Y, Kumanohoso T, Yoshifuku S, Matsukida K, Koriyama C, Kisanuki A, Minagoe S, Levine RA, Tei C. Isolated annular dilatation does not usually cause important functional mitral regurgitation: comparison between patients with lone atrial fibrillation and those with idiopathic or ischemic cardiomyopathy. J Am Coll Cardiol. 2002;39:1651–6.
30. Oki T, Fukuda N, Iuchi A, Tabata T, Yamada H, Fukuda K, et al. Possible mechanisms of mitral regurgitation in dilated hearts: a study using transesophageal echocardiography. Clin Cardiol. 1996;19:639–43.
31. Comin J, Manito N, Roca J, Castells E, Esplingas E. Functional mitral regurgitation: physiopathology and impact of medical therapy and surgical techniques for left ventricle reduction. Rev Esp Cardiol. 1999;52: 512–20.
32. Bolling SF, Pagani FD, Deeb GM, Bach DS. Intermediate-term outcome of mitral reconstruction in cardiomyopathy. J Thorac Cardiovasc Surg. 1998;115: 381–8.
33. Chandraratna PA, Aranow WS. Mitral valve ring in normal vs dilated left ventricle: cross-sectional echocardiographic study. Chest. 1981;79:152–4.
34. Bulkley BH, Roberts WC. Dilatation of the mitral annulus: a rare cause of mitral regurgitation. Am J Med. 1975;59:457–63.
35. He S, Lemmon JD, Weston MW, Jensen MO, Levine RA, Yoganathan AP. Mitral valve compensation for annular dilatation: in vitro study into the mechanisms of functional mitral regurgitation with an adjustable annulus model. J Heart Valve Dis. 1999;8:294–302.
36. Braile DM, Ardito RV, Pinto GH, Santos JL, Zaiantchick M, Souza DR. Plástica mitral. Rev Bras Circ Cardiovasc. 1990;5:86–98.
37. Hueb AC, Jatene FB, Moreira LFP, Pomerantzeff PM, Kallás E, de Oliveira SA. Ventricular remodelling and mitral valve modifications in dilated cardiomyopathy: new insights from anatomic study. J Thorac Cardiovasc Surg. 2002;124:1216–24.
38. Kunzelman KS, Cochran RP, Verrier ED, Eberhart RC. Anatomic basis for mitral valve modeling. J Heart Valve Dis. 1994;3:491–6.
39. Perloff JK, Roberts WC. The mitral apparatus: functional anatomy of mitral regurgitation. Circulation. 1972;46:227–39.
40. Brock RC. The surgical and pathological anatomy of the mitral valve. Br Heart J. 1952;14:489–513.
41. Cosgrove DM, Arcidi JM, Rodriguez L, Stewart WJ, Powell K, Thomas JD. Initial experience with the Cosgrove-Edwards annuloplasty system. Ann Thorac Surg. 1995;60:499–504.
42. Camilleri L, Filaire M, Repossini A, Legault B, Eder V, Fleury JP, et al. Mitral annuloplasty with a flexible linear reducer. J Card Surg. 1995;10:99–103.
43. Salati M, Scrofani R, Santoli C. Posterior pericardial annuloplasty: a physiological correction? Eur J Cardiothorac Surg. 1991;5:226–9.
44. Kono T, Sabbah H, Rosman H, Alam M, Jaffri S, Goldstein S. Left ventricular shape is the primary determinant of functional mitral regurgitation in heart failure. J Am Coll Cardiol. 1972;20:1594–8.
45. Wenk JF, Zhang Z, Cheng G, Malhotra D, Acevedo-Bolton G, Burger M, Suzuki T, Saloner DA, Wallace AW, Guccione JM, Ratcliffe MB. First finite element model of the left ventricle with mitral valve: insights into ischemic mitral regurgitation. Ann Thorac Surg. 2010;89:1546–53.
46. Corin WJ, Monrad ES, Murakami T, Nonogi H, Hess OM, Krayenbuehl HP. The relationship of afterload to ejection performance in chronic mitral regurgitation. Circulation. 1987;76:59–67.

47. Enriquez-Sarano M, Rossi A, Seward JB, Bailey KR, Tajik AJ. Determinants of pulmonary hypertension in left ventricular dysfunction. J Am Coll Cardiol. 1997; 29:153–9.
48. Bursi F, Enriquez-Sarano M, Jacobsen SJ, Roger VL. Mitral regurgitation after myocardial infarction: a review. Am J Med. 2006;119:103–12.
49. Carabello BA. Ischemic mitral regurgitation and ventricular remodeling. J Am Coll Cardiol. 2004;43: 384–5.
50. Prucz RB, Weiss ES, Patel ND, Nwakanma LU, Shah AS, Conte JV. The impact of surgical ventricular restoration on mitral valve regurgitation. Ann Thorac Surg. 2008;86:726–35.
51. Menicanti L, DiDonat M, Castelvecchio S, RESTORE group, et al. Functional ischemic mitral regurgitation in anterior ventricular remodeling: results of surgical ventricular restoration with and without mitral repair. Heart Fail Rev. 2004;9:317–27.
52. Kaza A, Patel M, Fiser S, et al. Ventricular reconstruction results in improved left ventricular function and amelioration of mitral insufficiency. Ann Surg. 2002;235:828–32.
53. Lee S, Chang B, Youn Y, Kwak Y, Yoo K. Changes in left ventricular function and dimension after surgical ventricular restoration with or without concomitant mitral valve procedure. Circ J. 2007;71:1516–20.
54. Maxey TS, Reece TB, Ellman PI, et al. Coronary artery bypass with ventricular restoration is superior to coronary artery bypass alone in patients with ischemic cardiomyopathy. J Thorac Cardiovasc Surg. 2004;127:428–34.
55. Yu HY, Su MY, Liao TY, Peng HH, Lin FY, Tseng WY. Functional mitral regurgitation in chronic ischemic coronary artery disease: analysis of geometric alterations of mitral apparatus with magnetic resonance imaging. J Thorac Cardiovasc Surg. 2004;128:543–51.
56. Mickleborough LL, Merchant N, Ivanov J, Rao V, Carson S. Left ventricular reconstruction: early and late results. J Thorac Cardiovasc Surg. 2004;128:27–37.
57. Barletta G, Toso A, Del Bene R, Di Donato M, Sabatier M, Dor V. Preoperative and late postoperative mitral regurgitation in ventricular reconstruction: role of local left ventricular deformation. Ann Thorac Surg. 2006;82:2102–9.
58. Fantini F, Barletta G, Baroni M, et al. Quantitative evaluation of left ventricular shape in anterior aneurysm. Cathet Cardiovasc Diagn. 1993;28:295–300.
59. Sheehan FH, Stewart DK, Dodge HT, Mitten S, Bolson EL, Brown BG. Variability in the measurement of regional left ventricular wall from contrast angiograms. Circulation. 1983;68:550–9.
60. Kass DA, Traill TA, Altieri PI, Maugham WL. Abnormalities of dynamic ventricular shape change in patients with aortic and mitral valvular regurgitation: assessment by Fourier shape analysis and global geometric indexes. Circ Res. 1988;62:127–38.
61. Gibson DG, Brown DJ. Continuous assessment of left ventricular shape in man. Br Heart J. 1975;37:904–10.
62. Baroni M, Barletta G. Digital curvature estimation for left ventricular shape analysis. Image Vision Comput. 1992;10:485–94.
63. Glasson JR, Komeda M, Daughters GT, et al. Most ovine mitral annular 3-D size reduction occurs before ventricular systole and is abolished with ventricular pacing. Circulation. 1997;96 Suppl 2:115–23.
64. Menicanti L, Di Donato M, Frigiola A, Buckberg G, Santambrogio C, Ranucci M, Santo D, RESTORE Group. Ischemic mitral regurgitation: intraventricular papillary muscle imbrication without mitral ring during left ventricular restoration. J Thorac Cardiovasc Surg. 2002;123:1041–50.
65. Parachuri VR, Adhyapak SM, Kumar P, Setty R, Rathod R, Shetty DP. Ventricular restoration by linear endoventricular patchplasty and linear repair. Asian Cardiovasc Thorac Ann. 2008;16:401–6.
66. Kasper EK, Agema WR, Hutchins GM, Deckers JW, Hare JM, Baughman KL. The causes of dilated cardiomyopathy: a clinicopathologic review of 673 consecutive patients. J Am Coll Cardiol. 1994;23:586–90.

Index

V R. Parachuri, S.M. Adhyapak, *Ventricular Geometry in Post-Myocardial Infarction Aneurysms*,
DOI 10.1007/978-1-4471-2861-8, © Springer-Verlag London 2012

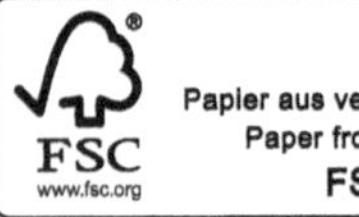

MIX
Papier aus verantwortungsvollen Quellen
Paper from responsible sources
FSC® C105338

If you have any concerns about our products,
you can contact us on
ProductSafety@springernature.com

In case Publisher is established outside the EU,
the EU authorized representative is:
Springer Nature Customer Service Center GmbH
Europaplatz 3, 69115 Heidelberg, Germany

Printed by Libri Plureos GmbH
in Hamburg, Germany